THE CLINICAL AND PROJECTIVE USE OF THE BENDER-GESTALT TEST

ABOUT THE AUTHOR

Eugene X. Perticone, Ed.D. (Rutgers) has conducted a private practice in psychotherapy and psychological assessment since 1971. A licensed psychologist, he was, for twenty-four years, a professor at the State University of New York at Oswego where he taught graduate courses in projective techniques, clinical assessment, personality theory, and adjustment. He has also worked as a psychologist in schools, was Director of Research and Evaluation for a comprehensive mental health facility, and served as a consultant psychological examiner for the New York State Department of Social Services. He is senior author of *The Mosaic Technique in Personality Assessment: A Practical Guide,* and he has lectured widely on that technique and the Bender-Gestalt Test. A recipient of the Graduate Research Award from the New Jersey Psychological Association, he is a member of the American Psychological Association, a fellow of the Society for Personality Assessment, a member of the Society for Clinical and Experimental Hypnosis, and he has been certified as an Approved Consultant by the American Society of Clinical Hypnosis.

THE CLINICAL AND PROJECTIVE USE OF THE BENDER-GESTALT TEST

By

EUGENE X. PERTICONE, ED.D.

Professor Emeritus
State University of New York, College at Oswego
Oswego, New York

Foreword by

John B. Ruskowski, Ph.D.

State University of New York, College at Oswego
Oswego, New York

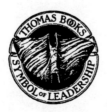

CHARLES C THOMAS · PUBLISHER, LTD.
Springfield · Illinois · U.S.A.

Published and Distributed Throughout the World by
CHARLES C THOMAS • PUBLISHER, LTD.
2600 South First Street
Springfield, Illinois 62794-9265

©1998 by CHARLES C THOMAS • PUBLISHER, LTD.
ISBN 0-398-06834-8 (cloth)
ISBN 0-398-06835-6 (paper)

Library of Congress Catalog Card Number: 97-43203

With THOMAS BOOKS *careful attention is given to all details of manufacturing
and design. It is the Publisher's desire to present books that are satisfactory as to their
physical qualities and artistic possibilities and appropriate for their particular use.*
THOMAS BOOKS *will be true to those laws of quality that assure a good name
and good will.*

Printed in the United States of America

SM-R-3

Library of Congress Cataloging-in-Publication Data

Perticone, Eugene X.
    The clinical and projective use of the Bender-Gestalt test/ by
Eugene X. Perticone; foreword by John B. Ruskowski.
p.   cm.
    Includes bibliographical references and index.
    ISBN 0-398-06834-8 (cloth).   ISBN 0-398-06835-6 (paper)
    1. Bender-Gestalt Test. 2. Personality assessment.
        I. Title.
RC473.B46P47 1998
616. 89'075--dc21   97-43203
                                                            CIP

For Freddie

FOREWORD

Carl Jung (1954) wrote, "Theories in psychology are the very devil. It is true that we need certain points of view for orienting and heuristic value, but they should always be regarded as mere auxiliary concepts that can be laid aside at any time" (p. 7). While we will always construct theories and test hypotheses in order to better understand the intricate workings of the mind, we must also remember that it is the human being, and not the theory itself, that is the goal of our understanding. Jung's statement seems to be warning us not to let our theories and our empirical derivations restrict our vision or our understanding of the true richness of any individual's experience. In the present volume, *The Clinical and Projective Use of the Bender-Gestalt Test*, Dr. Perticone opens a fresh, and eminently practical new window which enables the clinician to build upon the rich empirical history of this instrument. He offers an expanded view of the measure's potential utility, complementing familiar approaches with additional, projective applications that offer a highly efficient, useful, yet probing method for deepening one's understanding of the personal psychological experience of the test-taker.

Perhaps a reflection of our increasingly legalistic times, the literature in personality appraisal, for the past twenty years or so, has shown a strong bias toward refining or developing theoretical models and establishing empirical bases for the defensibility of tests and assessment practices. To be sure, strides have been made in those areas as well as in the areas of culture and gender fairness. An unfortunate effect, however, is that there has been a dearth of truly groundbreaking work in projective approaches to personality appraisal that has been both conceptually sophisticated and practical. Yet the blending of these two elements is precisely what Dr. Perticone has achieved in the present volume.

"Bender-Gestalt" and "groundbreaking work" are terms that have rarely been closely linked since Elizabeth Koppitz' (1964) book was published over thirty years ago. After all, clinicians already know the

Bender-Gestalt, don't they? Most are certainly familiar with empirically-based applications of this test in screening for neurological impairment and emotional difficulties. However, for those who are willing to accept that all behavior, including test-taking behavior, is psychologically meaningful, Dr. Perticone's clinical reasoning and case examples enable the reader to see and appreciate the untapped richness that is always present in the Bender-Gestalt. Furthermore, by adding Free-Association and Selective-Association phases to the task, additional data are elicited which, when integrated with the material generated by the Traditional approach, make it strikingly clear that very specific information about adjustment and personality is encoded in one's reproductions of the Bender-Gestalt designs and in the spontaneous and elicited verbalizations that are associated with them.

While clinicians can often sense that more is being communicated by an individual's test-taking behavior than is consciously intended, it is sometimes difficult to grasp and to organize these potential meanings. In his presentation of the projective use of the Bender-Gestalt, Dr. Perticone brings together his own extensive clinical experience, a rich understanding of personality dynamics, and his astute powers of observation. To these, he adds his remarkable ability to organize and express his procedures and methods for arriving at insights in an extremely cogent and practical way. The result is a truly valuable guide that will enable the skillful clinician to glean many useful projective hypotheses from the Bender-Gestalt record and to broaden his or her thinking about the potential applications of this familiar and ubiquitous instrument.

The Clinical and Projective Use of the Bender-Gestalt Test will not be the primary reference book for those practitioners who are constantly called upon to show statistical "proof" of their findings in order to validate their methods. This is a resource for people who work with people, where, Jung cautions, our theories may be the starting point, but must not be allowed to constrain the scope of our exploration. The uniqueness of each individual demands understanding rather than mere classification, and in the approach illustrated in this volume, the clinician's own knowledge of human dynamics and his or her skills of observation come to the fore. Dr. Perticone courageously discusses the roles of unconscious processes and clinical intuition in arriving at projective hypotheses. Yet, as a safeguard against mere conjecture masquerading as insight, he repeatedly returns to the principle of internal consistency and the use of collateral sources of information as means of supporting, elaborating, revising or discarding hypotheses.

This is a volume that will be appreciated by virtually anyone involved in personality appraisal, whether an experienced user of the Bender-Gestalt or a clinician-in-training. The reader will find Dr. Perticone's presentation of the expanded use of this instrument to be both stimulating and worthwhile. Veteran users will be able to add to the depth and richness of their findings based upon administration of the Bender, with little additional investment of time. Those who are just learning to appreciate the principles and subtleties of projective psychology will not find a more straightforward, clearly articulated introduction to fundamental concepts of projection in general and the projective use of the Bender-Gestalt Test in particular. The ample descriptions and discussions of interpretive features of the Bender drawings are further supplemented with over eighty selected illustrations.

It is gratifying to see this significant, new work in projective assessment which truly challenges and enables diagnosticians and psychotherapists to expand their present knowledge and practice in the use of the Bender-Gestalt. At the same time, this work helps to redirect attention toward both the importance of, and the possibility of, understanding the unique experience of each human being. Dr. Perticone invites readers to suspend preconceived notions about perceived limitations of the Bender-Gestalt, about projective assessment generally, and about the role of unconscious processes, while he guides them through a provocative, persuasive, and highly practical exploration of this "well-known" test.

JOHN B. RUSKOWSKI

REFERENCES

Jung, C. G. (1954). *The development of personality.* Princeton, NJ: Princeton University Press.

Koppitz, E. M. (1964). *The Bender-Gestalt Test for young children.* New York: Grune & Stratton.

---

[1] Jung, C. G. (1954). *The development of personality.* Copyright 1954 by Princeton University Press. Renewed 1984.

PREFACE

In the thirty-five years during which the author has used the Bender Visual-motor Gestalt Test in his clinical practice, he has consistently been impressed by its fruitfulness in providing a range of important information about a test subject and by its convenience as a diagnostic tool. It is extremely easy to administer, it takes a relatively short amount of time to complete, and it may be used alone or it can readily be included in any test battery. More importantly, in his clinical practice, it has not only been used as a measure of perceptual-motor development and competence, but as a convenient and wonderfully helpful means of assessing personality dynamics and functioning. It is the latter application that this book will emphasize.

The Bender Visual-motor Gestalt Test has long been used as a projective method, and numerous articles, chapters, and even longer works have been written about its value in this regard. In the current book, the attempt is made to (1) describe a method to increase the scope of the test subject's performance so that both verbal and nonverbal behaviors may be observed and (2) demonstrate an approach to generating clinically useful hypotheses about what the observed behaviors may signify about the person as an active and experiencing being.

In this book, the author demonstrates the importance of the parallel communications that are constantly being presented by the test subject, both verbally and nonverbally. Guidelines are provided to assist the psychological examiner in recognizing such communications and interpreting them dynamically. In addition, the author suggests that each of the individual Bender-Gestalt designs has the *potential* to symbolize a specific area of internal or external experience and that the symbolism may be anticipated, again potentially, to be similar for many, or even most, of the subjects who take the test. This is not to imply, however, that the symbolic pull of the designs is necessarily exactly as suggested for every test subject or that the designs may not hold additional symbolic meanings for certain individuals as well.

Nevertheless, the symbolic interpretations that are offered have proven to be so practically helpful and accurate in clinical work that it is believed they warrant consideration by those examiners who wish to get more out of a technique that is already being used, but with a different focus of attention. Also of interest is the fact that the method being advocated has been taught by the author to numerous psychologists-in-training as well as to many professionals already in the field, in both cases with very gratifying results. It is because of the successful application of this particular projective approach by those who employ it that it was decided to present the rationale and method in book form.

It is sincerely hoped that the personality assessment concepts that are presented will be considered with an open mind. Above all, the reader is encouraged to experiment with the expanded use of the Bender-Gestalt Test to see firsthand the wealth of interpretive material which will be made available to the astute clinical observer.

The detailed examples and "case presentations" that are used to illustrate the concepts and techniques of the expanded testing approach to be described are simulations of the kinds of responses and behaviors that are typically encountered in the clinical context. This book is essentially designed to be instructional in its organization and content. It is not intended to be a collection of case studies.

EUGENE X. PERTICONE

ACKNOWLEDGMENTS

The author wishes to express his gratitude to the many teachers and colleagues who have contributed so much to the development of his appreciation for the utility of projective psychology in clinical practice. The extent to which this frame of reference has helped him to understand people, to develop empathy for them, and to be of practical assistance when it was sought has been very great indeed.

Special thanks are extended to Leonard Blank, Ph.D., my clinical instructor and mentor at Rutgers-The State University, who skillfully taught the importance of carefully observing the living person, and not just his or her test responses, and to appreciate the indirect and subtle messages that are unconsciously communicated by the individual in the assessment situation.

Thanks also are due to Kay Sperry Showers who long ago stimulated the author to consider a potentially broader utility for the Bender-Gestalt Test and who demonstrated both its accuracy and value in personality assessment applications.

CONTENTS

LIST OF FIGURES

THE CLINICAL AND PROJECTIVE USE OF THE BENDER-GESTALT TEST

Part 1

QUANTITATIVE AND QUALITATIVE PERSPECTIVES ON THE BENDER-GESTALT TEST

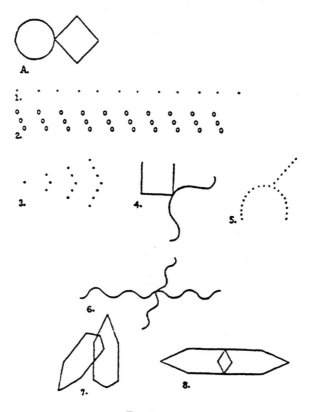

Figure 1

The Bender-Gestalt Designs. Reproduced from A *Visual Motor Gestalt Test and Its Clinical Use* by Lauretta Bender, copyright and distributed by the American Orthopsychiatric Association, Inc. Reproduced by permission.

Chapter 1

INTRODUCTION

A BRIEF RETROSPECTIVE

In 1938, Lauretta Bender published a monograph in which she described a framework and rationale for interpreting the attempts made by subjects to reproduce a series of sequentially presented geometric line drawings (Figure 1). The test was easy to administer, required relatively little time to complete, and enabled the examiner to observe directly the unique manner in which the task was carried out. Additionally, it resulted in a permanent visual record which facilitated analysis and categorization of the test subject's perceptual-motor responses.

That this pioneering work has been of practical as well as theoretical significance is attested to by the fact that the test which now bears Bender's name has become one of the most widely-used clinical measures of its type, with assessment applications having been demonstrated in a number of distinct, but interrelated areas of perceptual-motor functioning. Of course, Bender's method and the various applications that have been devised for it have subsequently been the focus of considerable research activity. Some studies have investigated the ability of the test to distinguish between various clinical and nonclinical groups while other studies have attempted to ascertain and operationalize performance standards that could be correlated with specific age or maturational levels. For summaries of both the clinical populations that have been researched and the efficacy of the various scoring and interpretive criteria that have been utilized, the reader is referred to the excellent reviews to be found in Tolor and Schulberg (1963) and Tolor and Brannigan (1980).

QUANTITATIVE AND QUALITATIVE INTERPRETATION

As might be expected, reliability and validity issues have been of central importance in many of the studies that have been published to date. Relatively fewer papers have attempted to demonstrate the ways in which Bender-Gestalt[1] performance can contribute to the clinician's understanding of the specific personality processes that are characteristic of the individual test subject or how those processes are related to his or her subjective experience or to the external manifestations of that experience, e.g., interpersonal behavior, ego-defensive operations, etc.

The present writer wishes to make clear that he acknowledges the value of the various quantitative systems that have been devised for categorizing and interpreting Bender-Gestalt performance. The developmental scoring system of Koppitz (1964; 1975), for example, has been shown to be a highly effective means of assessing perceptual-motor readiness for learning in school age youngsters, and is probably one of the more widely-used applications of the test at this time. Similarly, the demonstrated efficacy of the Bender-Gestalt Test in eliciting signs that may be indicative of neurological impairment or brain dysfunction (Klatskin, McNamara, Shaffer, & Pincus, 1972; Koppitz, 1962; Kramer & Penwick, 1966; Lacks & Newport, 1980) makes it highly likely that it will continue to be included in diagnostic batteries that are used when the presence of organicity is suspected in either children or adults.

In the present work, however, an attempt is made to show how qualitative analysis may be employed to complement, and not replace, the quantitative approaches to assessment that are presently emphasized in clinical work. The term *qualitative,* in this case, refers to the examiner's systematic observation and interpretation of the manner in which the test subject expresses his or her uniqueness, both verbally and nonverbally, in all aspects of the response to the test. This contrasts sharply with the more formal approaches to Bender-Gestalt interpretation in which the clinician's primary task is to calculate the quantitatively defined degree of accuracy (or inaccuracy) achieved by the test subject in the reproduction of the nine designs in order that a diagnostic classification can be made.

RATIONALE POR THE QUALITATIVE APPROACH

In the qualitative approach, clinical attention is directed not only to any inaccuracy occurring in the reproduction of a design that may constitute a scoreable error,[2] but also to *what the error itself seems to communicate about the test subject.* To illustrate, Figure 2.1 and Figure 2.2 show reproductions of Bender-Gestalt Design A by two different individuals. In each case, it readily may be seen that an error in size has occurred. Using a developmental scoring system such as that of Koppitz (1964), for example, each test subject can be assigned an error tally of one point that eventually will become part of an aggregate score for all the errors that occur in the reproductions of the nine Bender-Gestalt Designs. Once this quantitative determination has been made, i.e., ascertaining the presence or absence of an operationally defined error, the examiner's task with Design A may be considered to be complete.

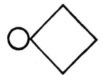

Figure 2.1

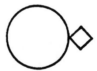

Figure 2.2

Qualitatively, however, the interpretative work has just begun. This is because the examiner now shifts to the projective frame of reference that assumes that *no psychological event occurs capriciously or accidentally, but on the contrary is the specific and meaningful outcome of a number of interacting events or conditions that already have occurred or are presently occurring within the psyche.* Included here are prior-existing drive-states, affects, and various defensive operations, albeit internal or unconscious ones. For the examiner trained to think in terms of the qualitative approach, the assumption in the case of either of the reproductions shown in Figure 2.1 and 2.2, therefore, will be that the error that has been made is in some way meaningful and that it reflects a subjective experiential state or personality dynamic present within the individual at the time the drawing was made.

Why, the examiner may speculate, was it the circle (or alternatively, the square) in particular that was made disproportionately large?

After all, there are two discreet elements that comprise the gestalt of Design A, and presumably either could have been the recipient of the extra energy required to increase the size of that element. Furthermore, what might the circle (or alternatively, the square) consciously or unconsciously symbolize for the test subject that would render it worthy of such increased energy expenditure? Or, if these questions are considered together, what drive, feeling, or attitude might the test subject be attempting to convey by enlarging one part of the design and, in effect, diminishing the relative size of the other? The present author has found that the seeking of answers to such questions can lead to very relevant and useful information about a test subject's psychodynamics that would not be revealed by the assigning of the error score alone.

By approaching the interpretation of the Bender-Gestalt Test from *both* quantitative *and* qualitative perspectives, the psychological examiner obtains a more complete picture of the test subject as a real and unique individual, as well as a member of a clinical or normative reference group. Thus, not only may the individual be diagnosed as being perceptually impaired, for example, but inferences may be drawn about how this person feels, what significant conflicts are being experienced, whether interpersonal contact is sought or avoided, and whether or not the perceptual impairment may be the result of emotional, rather than organic, factors. Hypotheses of this type are, of course, of special interest to clinicians who hope to do more to help the individual than simply render an opinion as to which clinical group or maturational level he or she should be assigned.

This book, then, emphasizes the importance of the psychodynamic factors that may have an influence on both the test subject's perception of the separate stimulus figures and his or her ability to reproduce them accurately. These psychodynamics are largely unconscious and may be symbolically expressed through even the most subtle distortions in the reproductions. Unfortunately, since the records of maturationally normal subjects beyond the age of eleven typically yield a zero error score, according to the commonly used tabular systems, many examiners curtail their clinical observation and inferential reasoning and ignore the many nonscoreable, but nevertheless revealing, features that are actually present in the design reproductions and can be understood as expressions of the individual's psychodynamics.

From this perspective, then, it is possible to interpret every record, even when no scoreable errors have been made. Viewed in this way, the Bender-Gestalt Test can be considered a *general measure of personality functioning.* It can be employed, as Lerner (1972) points out, as a tool that assists the examiner to understand what the test subject is experiencing and then to infer how he or she may behave in other life situations. Utilized in this way, the Bender-Gestalt becomes a means of assessment that can be exploited effectively in a much wider role than is commonly the case. In the practice of psychotherapy, for instance, it becomes a rapid and surprisingly revealing source of hypotheses concerning the client's personality functioning that can be tested at any time during a treatment session and that can be used in the initial planning of tactics and strategies that will be appropriate for the more long-term treatment plan.

ENDNOTES

1. In this book, *Bender Visual-motor Gestalt Test, Bender-Gestalt Test,* or simply *Bender-Gestalt* will be used interchangeably.

2. Although various scoring systems have been suggested for assessing the accuracy of Bender-Gestalt reproductions (e.g., Pascal & Suttell, 1951; Clawson, 1962; Lacks, 1984), the *errors* referred to in this book will be defined by the operational criteria specified by Koppitz (1964).

Chapter 2

THE PSYCHODYNAMIC PERSPECTIVE

THE EXAMINATION EXPERIENCE

When approaching any testing situation, it may be assumed that stimulus generalization is occurring. That is, the test subject brings to the testing moment an extensive history of other experiences of having been evaluated. Evaluation of academic readiness often begins prior to entry into kindergarten, for example, and for the remainder of the child's school life, informal testing is routinely conducted year after year, in one classroom after another, in order to assess the extent to which the curriculum has been mastered. In addition, the child eventually is subjected to formal or psychometrically-based schoolwide testing programs that have been designed to determine achievement levels, academic aptitude, vocational interests, etc. Later in life, tests will be required in nonacademic settings as well, as when applying for a driver's license or in connection with some job applications.

Besides those formal occasions that are clearly recognized as "testing" situations, there are other encounters that are not necessarily defined as "being tested," but which are nevertheless experienced as such. A child being asked by a parent to display his or her hands after washing so that their degree of cleanliness may be determined is just one of the many examples of one's performance being evaluated with which most readers should be familiar.

In any event, it appears that the circumstance of being tested is a recurrent one that, in most cases, is likely to be experienced as anything but neutral. That is, how a person is categorized and/or responded to by others as a result of an evaluation procedure is often associated with specific emotional side effects. And while these may be neutral or even pleasant for some, observation suggests that for many persons the occasion of being tested results in some degree of tension and even anxiety. It is common, for instance, for certain individuals to suffer autonomic symptoms in anticipation of a test, while in some cases anxiety actually becomes so great that blocking will occur to the extent that the individual may actually be unable to perform, or may perform at a level well below that of which he or she is otherwise capable. Sarason, S. B., Davidson, K. S., Lighthall, P. P., Waite, R. R., and Ruebush, B. K. (1960), in their study of both general and test anxiety in children, conclude that the occasion of being tested is often noxious because it represents the prior experience of having been evaluated, for example, by parents, in other types of situations, and that such evaluations have frequently been associated with feelings of rejection, guilt, loss of self-esteem, or other threats to psychological security.

In light of such considerations, it seems reasonable to assume that stimulus generalization is also likely to occur when one is administered the Bender-Gestalt Test, and that some degree of psychological threat undoubtedly will be experienced by the test subject. It also follows that in response to such threat, both conscious and unconscious defenses will be mobilized in order to deal with the anxiety that can be expected to accompany it. To put it another way, the occasion of being examined with the Bender-Gestalt, as with any similar psychological assessment technique, provides an opportunity for the examiner to observe not only the test subject's specific productions when he or she is asked to copy the designs, but also to observe the qualitatively significant behaviors and performance characteristics from which can be inferred the person's experience of anxiety and the defenses that are being used to manage it.

THE STRIVING SELF AND PERSONALITY PROJECTION

Strivings that have been described as being central to the functioning of all human beings involve not only efforts to preserve physical safety, but also to maintain the perception of personal adequacy or self-esteem (Combs & Snygg, 1959). Whether considered to be rooted in biology, learned experience, or a combination of these factors, the relevant point is that all individuals continuously strive to satisfy both of these motives which may be described respectively as the need for security and the need to obtain the approval of self and/or others.

The position taken by the present author is that needs such as those identified above are incredibly strong and can be assumed to play some part, directly or indirectly, in virtually all goal-directed behavior. The presence of these needs is often easily recognized even by the casual observer as, for example, when one is watching the behavior patterns of children who are interacting in play, whether it be competitive or noncompetitive in nature. At other times, the external manifestations of such ego-strivings will be less obvious except in those instances where the observer has been trained to anticipate their existence and so remains specifically alert for the signs from which their presence may be deduced. As noted in an earlier work (Perticone & Tembeckjian, 1987), this is the type of process that underlies the efforts of the psychodynamically-oriented counselor or psychotherapist who constantly monitors not only the *literal content* of a client's verbalizations, but considers the *symbolic implications* of the words and phrases being used, as well as the numerous nonverbal communications and gestures that are so often laden with disguised personal meaning.

AN EXPANDED APPROACH TO THE BENDER-GESTALT TEST

In the material that follows, a three-phase technique for the administration of the Bender-Gestalt Test will be presented. The purpose of this approach is to obtain information beyond that commonly sought, in the quantitative scoring methods with which many examiners are already familiar, by including two additional phases that will emphasize the projective or qualitative perspective discussed above. By doing this, the Bender-Gestalt becomes a multidimensional assessment tool through which meaningful hypotheses may be generated about the individual's personality dynamics *as well as* his or her psychoneurological integrity and/or maturational level. The three phases of the expanded test administration are discussed in the next chapter under the headings of *The Traditional Procedure, The Free-Association Procedure,* and *The Selective-Association Procedure.*

Chapter 3

THE MULTIPHASE ADMINISTRATION

THE TRADITIONAL PROCEDURE

The first step in the administration of the expanded Bender-Gestalt follows guidelines similar to those that have been suggested by previous writers. Naturally, if a standardized scoring system is to be used for which quantitative norms are provided, for example, when using The Developmental Scoring System of Koppitz (1964), the specific directions for administration that are provided by the respective author should be followed exactly.

The present author proceeds in precisely that manner for test subjects below the age of ten. For older subjects, the following approach to administration is employed:

Assuming that adequate rapport has already been established, the test subject is given a sheet of 8 1/2 x 11 inch white paper that is unlined. (Mimeograph paper or paper with a similar surface texture is excellent for the purpose.) A sharpened Number Two pencil equipped with an eraser is also provided. Extra sheets of paper should be available on the table or other working surface and in easy reach of the person being tested. The test subject is then told that nine cards will be placed before him or her, and that each bears a design that is to be copied on the paper that has been provided. The examiner proceeds by placing the neatly stacked stimulus cards immediately above the paper, with Design A faceup at the top, saying:

> Here are the designs you are to copy. Make yours look just like the ones you see on each of these cards.

The test subject is allowed to reposition the cards if desired and to uncover the succeeding card as each drawing is completed. Questions that are raised should be answered only in general terms or by repeating the relevant portion of the original directions. For example, if asked, "Can I make them bigger?" or, "Do I need to draw all the dots?" the examiner may respond by pointing to the cards and saying, "Make yours look just like these." If the test subject inquires, "Can I use more than one piece of paper?" the response might be, "That's up to you." As much as practical, in other words, the examiner maintains ambiguity concerning the test subject's response choices for anything beyond the directions that were originally administered.

The examiner should generally remain silent while carefully observing the test subject's behavior that includes not only the drawing process, but all other verbal and nonverbal expressions as well. These are recorded as they occur whether they appear to relate specifically to the drawing process or not. The total time required to finish the nine designs is also noted and recorded. Upon completion of all the drawings, a testing-of-the-limits procedure may be employed at the examiner's discretion. Ordinarily this is done if (1) there is doubt about the test subject's awareness of errors or unusual features that have occurred in the reproductions or (2) it seems desirable to ascertain whether or not the test subject can reproduce the designs more accurately. However, unless there is such a clinically appropriate reason for doing so, an inquiry following this part of the test procedure is not advocated.

THE FREE-ASSOCIATION PROCEDURE

With the completion of the first phase of the administration, the-examiner removes the paper on which the designs have been drawn and puts it aside, thanking the test subject for having cooperated. The pencil and extra sheets of paper are also removed at this time. The examiner then collects the nine cards and places the stack face down on the table with Design A uppermost. The test subject is then told:

Now I have something else for you to do. I will again show you the designs, but this time I want you to use your imagination and tell me what each one reminds you of, or what it might represent.

The examiner hands Card A to the test subject and says:

For example, what does this design make you think of? What does it remind you of?"

If the test subject expresses uncertainty as to how to proceed, the examiner encourages with words such as:

Just use your imagination. When you do, the design will remind you of something. Go ahead. What comes to mind when you look at the design? What does it look like?

Having administered the directions, the examiner waits for the response which, when forthcoming, should be written down verbatim. The position in which the card is held should be noted for the respective associations. A notation should also be made of the test subject's initial reaction time, that is, the time elapsed between the presentation of the stimulus card and the response which is made to it. In this connection, the term *response* refers to the communication of the association itself, and not to preliminary remarks such as, "Oh, this is interesting," or, "Hmmm. Let me think about this one."

If only a single response is given for Card A, the examiner may ask, "Anything else?" This often leads to further associations that, if given, are to be recorded. If the test subject fails to provide an association to a particular design or says something like, "It doesn't remind me of anything," the examiner should encourage a further effort. Gently saying, "Use your imagination and just tell me whatever comes to mind," is often sufficient to elicit a response or to overcome the resistance to communicating a thought or image that, although not spoken, nonetheless may have been experienced.

At times, the test subject's specific associations will be vague or they may otherwise seem to be incomplete. In other instances, the examiner may intuit that a response has some clinically relevant implication or significance that would be worth exploring further. On occasions such as these, a cautious inquiry should be conducted. Examples of the inquiry procedure are demonstrated in the following interchanges:

(Associations to Card 7)

Subject: Reminds me of a carton with some milk. It's bulged on the bottom, and the one on the left is tipping over.
Examiner: You said, "bulged on the bottom." Explain that.
Subject: Bulged . . . Because it's ready to explode . . . Because it can't stand up anymore.

In this example, it was decided to inquire as to the test subject's choice of the word, *bulged*, since its meaning was not clear to the the examiner. In an attempt to clarify it, the subject attends less to the definition of the word, and projects instead the experience of tension or impulse that seems to be on the verge of being released.

(Associations to Card 3)

Subject: This looks like a tipped-over Christmas tree [spoken in a whisper].
Examiner: It looks like it's tipped over?
Subject: Yes. I guess I feel very sad when I look at it.

Here, it was thought that the association of the tree being tipped over, combined with the subdued nature of her verbal communication with the examiner, might symbolically express some experience of importance to the test subject. That this appears to be the case is supported by the personal reference made concerning the individual's affective experience.

Clearly, there can be no absolute rule as to when a test subject's response warrants inquiry. For the examiner experienced in assessing projection as it occurs in the testing situation or in the process of counseling, that determination will probably be made with relative ease. For the examiner less experienced in principles of projective psychology, an effort should be made to remain alert to the occurrence of vague language, the use of words with multiple meanings, e.g., punning words, or the use of words that are likely to be emotionally evocative for most people. In such cases, inquiry may be helpful since it provides opportunity for elaboration that can clarify the consciously intended meaning of the test subject's communication, and also because it forces the individual to encounter the potentially significant material that might otherwise be sidestepped.   When such an encounter is precipitated by the examiner's inquiry, several highly dynamic and interrelated processes are likely to be observed:

1. Further symbolic material may be presented.
2. Emotions may be expressed or otherwise revealed, e.g., through autonomic activity.
3. Defensive operations may become much more apparent thereby making it easier for the examiner to gauge the degree of threat that is being experienced as well as the nature and effectiveness of the defenses used to cope with that threat.

While a case is being made for the importance of the inquiry in the second phase of the Bender-Gestalt administration, it is probably better to underemphasize this procedure than to overemphasize its use until sufficient experience has been accrued by the examiner. This is because it is crucially important to minimize the risk of establishing a set in the test subject's mind as to what type of association to the stimulus figures might be considered appropriate.

THE SELECTIVE-ASSOCIATION PROCEDURE

In the second, or Free-Association, phase of the test administration, the examiner's intent is to elicit verbal associations to the Bender-Gestalt designs in a manner that allows the test subject considerable freedom to respond on the basis of his or her unique perceptions and dynamics. For this reason, directions are given in as general or ambiguous a fashion as possible so that the subject will know how to proceed, but not what content to produce.

In the third, or Selective-Association, phase, however, the purpose is to provide the opportunity for further personality projection, but this time with the examiner exercising more influence over the direction of the test subject's associations. To accomplish this, the examiner says to the subject:

That was fine. Now we will do the final portion of the test.

The examiner then arranges the nine stimulus cards face up before the test subject in three rows of three each and says:

I would like you to use your imagination again. This time I want you to look carefully at all of the designs and tell me which one you like the best.

The examiner observes to be sure that all of the designs are being considered. When a response is given, either verbally or by pointing, the examiner records the number of the stimulus card and any comments that are made and continues:

Now look at all of the designs again, but this time tell me which one you like the least.

Once again, the test subject's total behavior pattern is observed, and the response is recorded when given. The examiner then says:

Now really stretch your imagination and tell me which one makes you think most of your mother.

After the response and any accompanying comments have been noted, the examiner asks:

And which design makes you think most of your father?

When a record of the ensuing response is made, the examiner continues:

And which one makes you think most of yourself?

While the test may be concluded following the response to this question, the examiner instead may choose to elicit further associations that could be clinically relevant. If the test subject has a spouse, for example, an association to a particular design might be requested for *husband* or *wife*. Associations also may be elicited for other persons, e.g., *brother, sister, boss, teacher,* or for anything else deemed to be relevant to the test subject's life.

In addition to recording the actual associations, other significant observations should be noted. Ancillary comments are of interest, for example, as are changes in tone or volume, unusual motor activity, dramatic facial expressions, and signs of nervousness such as nail-biting. A notation should also be made when there is an extended delay between the examiner's instruction and the test subject's verbal response.

Part 2

PROJECTIVE INTERPRETATION
OF THE
BENDER-GESTALT TEST

Chapter 4

THE PROCESS OF
CLINICAL INTERPRETATION

GENERAL CONSIDERATIONS

In the discussion of the expanded or multiphase administration of the Bender-Gestalt Test that was presented above, the importance of observing a variety of subject behaviors was stressed. Such observations, it was explained, should include not only the subject's specific verbal responses to the directions administered by the examiner, but also should encompass the many ancillary comments and behaviors that accompany them. To consider the subject's productions without attending to the total manner in which they are delivered is to ignore the very aspects of individuality that reveal the subject as an actual person rather than as a quantified abstraction of one. The clinical focus of the examiner, therefore, will be broad in range. In the multiphase administration of the Bender-Gestalt Test, the examiner's attention will be directed to:

1. The actual drawings that have been rendered by the test subject.
2. The verbal associations elicited by the examiner in connection with the drawings.
3. The ancillary comments and utterances spontaneously made that in some instances appear to be pertinent to the actual productions and in other instances are seemingly irrelevant to them.
4. Nonverbal behaviors, such as finger-tapping, or indications of autonomic activity, such as blushing, that suggest specific affects are occurring.

QUANTITATIVE ANALYSIS OF THE PROTOCOL

When the test subject has copied the nine stimulus figures, the examiner has a permanent visual record that permits a careful analysis of the work done. As indicated earlier, the first step, that assumes primary importance when adults suspected of organicity or when young children are being tested, is to evaluate the "correctness" of the separate design reproductions. This phase necessitates close observation, that is, scrutiny, of the subject's renderings of the designs in order to determine whether or not they contain errors as operationally defined according to the scoring system that is being used. Once the error score has been determined, the quantitative interpretation can be made by referring to the appropriate norms tables for that system. Hypotheses can be generated, for instance, related to the test subject's perceptual-motor functioning as it is likely to affect school achievement or job performance or as evidence of the presence of organic involvement, etc. Once the normative status of the subject has been considered, the examiner is ready for qualitative or projective analysis.

INITIAL ASPECTS OF PROJECTIVE ANALYSIS

Projective interpretation, that is the focus of this book, begins with the evaluation of the subject's Bender-Gestalt record and extends to his or her response to the testing experience as a whole. This includes analysis of each of the following:

1. The subject's manner of responding to the examiner and the directions that are provided.
2. Arrangement of the designs and the use of space on the paper.
3. Unusual or distinctive design or protocol features, other than scoreable errors.
4. Spontaneous behaviors of the examinee, especially those occurring while designs are being drawn or while associations are being made to them.
5. Verbal associations to the stimulus figures.

Naturally, the number and variety of behaviors or signs apparent in each of these areas that will be considered to be interpretively important will vary with the experience, sophistication, and intuitiveness of the examiner. However, for purposes of this book, it will be useful to assume that *each and every design and protocol feature as well as every instance of the subject's behavior will have some level of potentially relevant meaning*. That is, each bit of verbal and nonverbal behavior will reflect some aspect of the subject's personality structure, dynamics, or development, and such information can contribute to an overall understanding of the individual being assessed.

The Response to the Examiner

It is important to bear in mind that each part of the Multiphase Administration constitutes an opportunity to observe the test subject's manner of adjusting to a new performance situation. It follows, then, that the examiner should focus not only on the perceptual accuracy of each drawing made by the subject in Phase One (Traditional Procedure) or the reasonableness of the associations that are made during Phase Two (Free-Association Procedure) and Phase Three (Selective-Association Procedure), but an effort should be made to deduce the more general indicators of adjustment that may be characteristic of the subject, and are not peculiar to the Bender-Gestalt Test alone.

Attitudes such as cooperativeness and self-confidence, for example, may be inferred from the subject's interpersonal manner and the smoothness and tempo of responding, while traits such as impulsivity or reflectiveness, cautiousness or recklessness may be deduced from the speed of responding and sometimes from verbal comments that accompany the act of drawing. Requesting further instructions of the examiner prior to beginning the task, for instance, may imply a preference for following, rather than leading, others when in new interpersonal situations. In a similar way, a subject who asks for permission, e.g., "Can I draw it sideways?" may be indicating more than a possible difficulty with spatial relations. In this instance, additional hypotheses might concern the subject's need to restructure interpersonal situations on his or her own terms before feeling safe enough to respond, or the request for permission may be a subconscious admission that what the test subject reveals will be done evasively or in a way to make it appear different than it actually is, i.e., "sideways." It also seems likely that the test subject is revealing the tendency to feel dependent on, or to be submissive to, authority figures. Of course, observations and hypotheses such as these will be strengthened if responses to subsequent Bender-Gestalt designs are accompanied by similar corroborative evidence.

Arrangement of the Designs

In reproducing the designs, the subject may arrange the individual drawings on the paper in a number of different ways. Placement may proceed in a highly sequential manner, for example, or in a fashion that seems to suggest that no plan was followed for their placement. Clawson (1962) hypothesizes that arrangement reflects an individual's intellectual approach. The present writer endorses this view, but emphasizes that one's intellectual approach, or cognitive style, as it is likely to be called today, represents a way of dealing with the world in general, and may specifically reflect the individual's characteristic way of defending the ego. For example, while a systematic arrangement of the designs suggests planning ability, it also may reflect the desire of the individual for consistency and predictability in his or her psychosocial world. By logical extension, then, the hypothesis is that subjects producing a very systematic arrangement of designs on the paper have a need to feel that they are in control in various life situations. And since much of life involves interacting with others, it follows that they are likely to be uncomfortable when interpersonal relations are ambiguous or when they are not sure of what is expected of them in the interpersonal context. The prominence of this need in a test subject's character structure is assumed to be proportionate to the effort that is expended to insure orderliness in the sequence of design placement. Figure 3 shows a record of this type. Here, the arrangement reflects perfectionism and a compulsive need for orderliness, traits that are likely to be consistent with the drawer's characteristic behavior in both work and social settings.

In some protocols, of course, arrangement of the designs may be less rigorously systematic, but still more or less sequential. The implication would be that while anticipation or ability to think ahead is indicated, the need to organize one's defenses around these traits is less compulsive in nature and that there may be greater tolerance for ambiguity in the psychosocial environment.

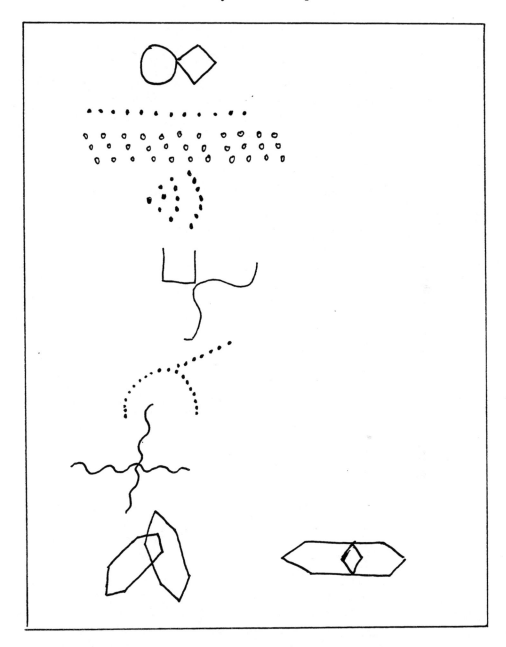

Figure 3

In other protocols, arrangement of the designs may reflect not only an absence of orderliness, but also what might appear to be a chaotic approach to placement of the drawings. In many such instances, the absence of sequence does not appear to be simply a function of developmental immaturity (as would be expected in very young children or

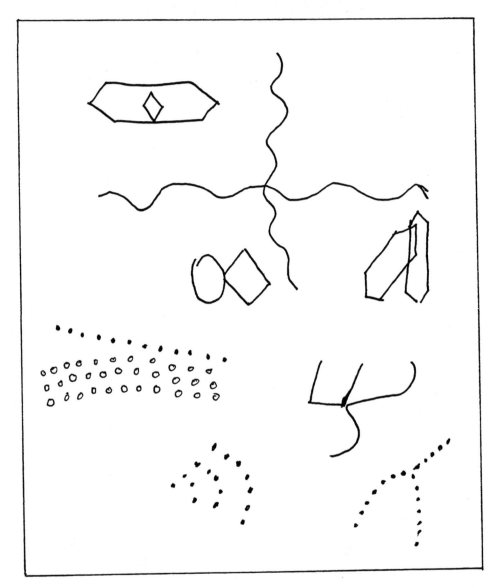

Figure 4

in the case of mental retardation), but instead may reflect reactions to the unpredictable inner promptings of the subject. This may indicate the character trait of impulsivity, i.e., the absence of reflection prior to responding to events, or in other instances may be the result of mental confusion.

Figure 4 illustrates a protocol typical of an impulsive older adolescent diagnosed as having a conduct disorder. Consistent with the lack

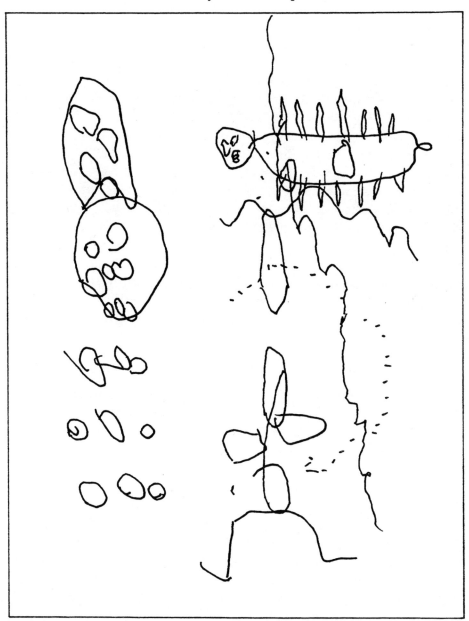

Figure 5

of planning that is suggested by the nonsequential, even disorderly, arrangement of the designs, is the brief amount of time required to complete the nine figures (one minute, 35 seconds).

Figure 5 represents a record that might have been produced by a confused subject who has been diagnosed as schizophrenic. Not only can placement of the designs be seen to be very disorderly, but the odd and unexpected elaborations that are present in the drawings appear to reflect an autistic process.

Utilization of Space

Another protocol feature that is felt to be of special importance relates to the portion of the sheet of paper used for the design reproductions, i.e., where on the page the designs are actually reproduced. Most subjects disperse their drawings over the entire sheet of paper. At times, however, the nine figures will be confined to the top or to the bottom only, or to the right or to the left only. The inevitable consequence of such consolidation of the drawings is that large portions of the paper will appear to be noticeably blank. While arrangements limited to a specific restricted area, such as right side as opposed to left side of the paper, may not reflect the identical personality tendency in all individuals, the resulting proximity of the drawings to each other often does seem to indicate a withdrawal tendency in the subject and/or the propensity for restricting self-expression in the psychosocial environment. In addition, two consolidated placements that appear to deserve particular clinical attention are those in which the designs seem to be suspended at the top of the page and those that seem to hug the bottom.

A tentative hypothesis to be considered with a markedly top placement is the presence of an active fantasy life, perhaps associated with high levels of aspiration. That the designs are compressed suggests, however, that the aspirations are in some way inhibited or are expressed in a passive, and possibly a passive-aggressive, manner (Figure 6). A conspicuous bottom placement, on the other hand, often seems to be associated with dependency and/or withdrawal, the latter tendency being especially likely if the figures are also small in size or drawn with very light pencil pressure. An example of bottom placement is shown in Figure 7.

A special instance of the unusual treatment of space occurs when a test subject utilizes both sides of a single sheet of paper to reproduce the designs or actually uses more than one sheet to complete them. In summarizing her research findings, Koppitz (1964) notes that using two or more sheets of paper, a behavior that she refers to as *expansiveness,* is not uncommon in children of preschool age, but that it could be associated with impulsiveness and acting-out tendencies in the case of older children, and recommends that the possibility of brain injury should be considered when it is observed in children of school age.

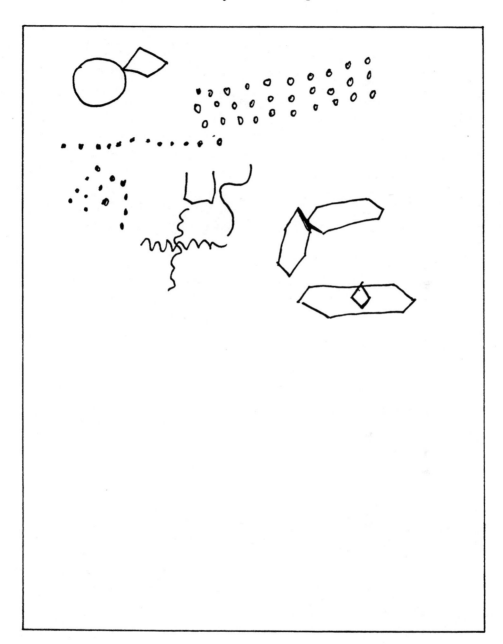

Figure 6

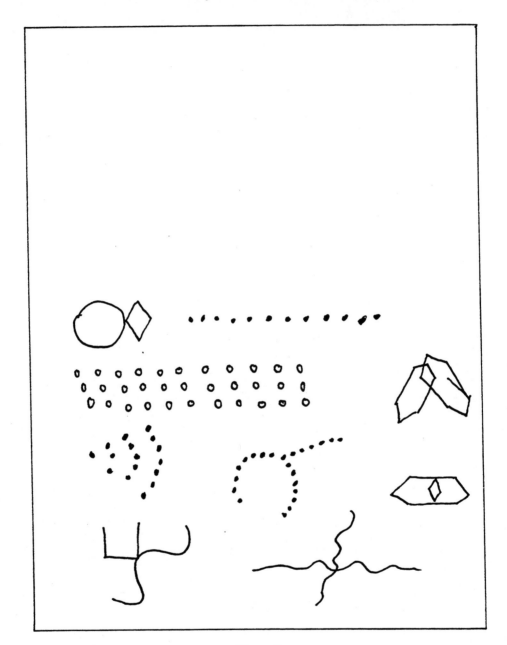

Figure 7

Specific Design Features

Numerous irregularities in the rendering of individual Bender-Gestalt designs have been reported in the literature to be diagnostically significant. Among the signs that have been investigated are features such as pencil pressure, closure difficulties, angulation difficulties, modification of circles or dots, overlapping drawings, changes in figure size, discrepancies in spatial orientation of the figures, unnecessary or bizarre elaborations, etc. Many of these individual signs, the hypotheses that are associated with them, and the supportive research citations are neatly summarized by Ogdon (1975) and by Gilbert (1978), and the Bender-Gestalt examiner should become familiar with them.

In an effort to differentiate between well-adjusted children and children with emotional difficulties, Koppitz (1964) investigated a number of such design or protocol features, ten of which were found to be useful enough to organize into a Scoring Manual for Emotional Indicators. The specific signs, or indicators, that she found to be significant, and the hypotheses she suggests for each can be summarized as follows:

Confused order of arrangement of the designs on the paper suggests mental confusion and planning difficulties; *wavy line* (change in direction of lines in Designs 1 or 2) may relate to emotional instability; *dashes* in place of circles (Design 2) suggests impulsivity; *large size* of figure as well as *expansion* (using two or more sheets of paper on which to copy the designs) may indicate an acting-out tendency; *overwork* of lines in part or all of a figure suggests aggressiveness or impulsiveness; *second attempt* at drawing a design connotes anxiety or impulsiveness; progressively *increasing size* of the circles or dots in Designs 1, 2, or 3 may reflect low frustration tolerance; and *small size* of figure and figures drawn with *fine line* point to timidity, shyness, and withdrawal characteristics.[1]

From a study of the research, Koppitz (1964) concludes that both individual emotional indicators and the total number of indicators present in a given record have diagnostic value, and that the total number of indicators in the record appears to be an index of the severity of the emotional disturbance. She also makes it clear that it is important for the examiner to bear in mind the fact that although individual indicators or signs may predict personality characteristics with some degree of accuracy, the presence of an indicator in itself does not necessarily warrant a diagnosis of emotional disturbance.

---

[1]From Koppitz, E. M. (1964). *The Bender Gestalt Test for Young Children.* Adapted by permission of Allyn and Bacon.

For anyone who has used the Bender-Gestalt test over time, it becomes obvious that the number of variations that may be found in reproductions of the stimulus figures is very great and may include types in addition to those listed above. Since no listing of signs can be considered to be definitive, the examiner must be prepared to recognize not only the deviations that have been mentioned, but any other unusual features that occur in the subject's drawings of the designs. In this connection, it seems appropriate to discuss several such features, some of which have already been mentioned, for which hypotheses that specifically pertain to personality functioning should routinely be considered. These include (1) circles being substituted for dots, (2) flattening and blunting of part or parts of a design, (3) workover of lines, and (4) occurrence of slope in the design that has been drawn. It should be kept in mind that these features, whether they constitute developmentally defined scoring errors or not, take on increased clinical significance as an index of personality functioning when they occur in the records of adolescents or adults.

Circles Substituted for Dots

The substitution of circles for dots is sometimes seen in the reproductions of Bender-Gestalt Designs 1, 3, and 5 (Figure 8). This is a fairly common occurrence in the drawings of young children and may be an index of developmental lag, depending on the age of the subject. It apparently does not carry significant weight as a diagnostic indicator of possible neurological impairment, however, until the age of seven in the case of Design 1 and until the age of nine in the case of Design 5 (Koppitz, 1964).

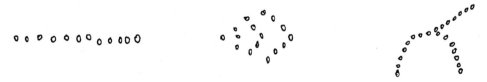

Figure 8

In terms of personality assessment, which is the main focus of the present book, the drawing of circles in the place of dots is often seen in the records of older subjects, including adolescents and adults, for whom the question of organicity is not a consideration. In such instances, this deviation appears to reflect immaturity and as such may represent some degree of fixation or regression within the character structure, usually in connection with a specific area or areas of actual life functioning. Behavioral manifestations of immaturity are likely to be seen, for example, in the conduct of interpersonal relations and the manner in which drives and impulses are typically managed. Specific hypotheses concerning the objects toward which such tendencies are expressed will be presented in Chapter 5 which deals with the symbolism of the individual Bender-Gestalt stimulus figures.

Flattening and Blunting

These terms refer to particular deviations that generally fall within the scoring category referred to as *distortion of shape*. They are mentioned separately here because they often appear to bear no relationship to organicity or physiological development, but will be found to have great projective value instead. That is to say, these deviations seem to possess particular symbolic significance, the interpretation of which can contribute much to the understanding of the personality dynamics and emotional adjustment of the individual being tested.

An example of flattening may be seen in Figure 9.1. Here, the circle portion of the Design A is drawn as an oval, i.e., it appears to be compressed. It is hypothesized that what is being communicated by the flattening is a sense of pressure or strong influence (probably interpersonal in nature) having been experienced to the extent that an individual has felt the need to restrict or otherwise change himself or herself in order to adjust to the power of another person or group of persons. A similar hypothesis would apply to the flattening of a hexagon in Design 7, an example of which is shown in Figure 9.2.

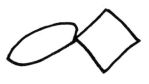

Figure 9.1

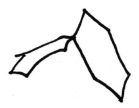

Figure 9.2

That the flattening of one of the elements in a design may suggest an individual who experiences substantial environmental pressure is often supported by the examiner's inquiry of the test subject. When questioned about such a deviation in the drawing of a Bender-Gestalt design, for example, subjects often will acknowledge the error with comments such as, "It looks like it's been squeezed."

Flattening also may occur in the examinee's reproduction of Design 6 (Figure 10). As will be elaborated later, this design appears to elicit projections of mood. When the amplitude of the individual curves, particularly the horizontal, is less than that of the curves in the actual stimulus figure, the interpretation is one of depressed mood, low energy level, or a tendency to inhibit expression of emotions.

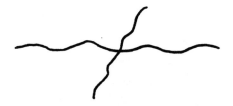

Figure 10

Inhibition of hostile impulses and the attempt to deny the existence of hostile feelings should also be considered strong possibilities when blunting of angles is noted. This is especially so when the angle or pointed part of one of the elements in a Bender-Gestalt design makes contact with a second element within the same design. Examples of this are shown in Figure 11.

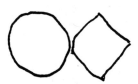

Figure 11

Workover of Lines

This category of response is essentially the same as that referred to as *overwork* or *reinforced line* by Koppitz (1964) in her discussion of emotional indicators in the Bender-Gestalt records of children. The term *workover* has been chosen for the present book in order to emphasize that the reworking of lines is being used as a *projective indicator* of the subject's experience rather than as an indicator to be summed with others in order to arrive at a diagnostic classification such as *emotional disturbance.*

Workover typically involves not only repetition of the pencil stroke when executing a drawing, but also pencil pressure that is greater than that exerted by the subject when completing other designs or different parts of the same design. The type of workover that is of particular clinical interest is that which occurs at the point where two separate, but complete, elements of a single design are expected to make contact with one another. This applies particularly to Designs A, 4, 6, 7, and 8. Examples of workover are shown in Figure 12.

The primary hypothesis to be considered when workover occurs in a Bender-Gestalt record is that a pronounced interpersonal conflict exists, usually between the test subject and a significant other. More rarely, however, it may be found, e.g., during counseling, that this drawing feature reflects instead an awareness of an intense conflict that exists between two other persons who have some close connection with the test subject. In either instance, the presence of reworked lines at the juncture of the separate design elements suggests that a state of tension is experienced by the individuals involved and that a strong emotional barrier exists between them.

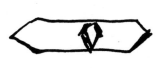 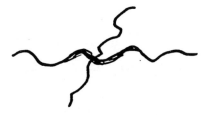

Figure 12

Slope

In many instances, Bender-Gestalt designs are drawn in such a manner that all or part of a design will be seen to slope in an upward or a downward direction. The term *slope* is used here since the deviation from the horizontal axis (represented by the right and left edges of the paper) often is not great enough to meet the criterion for scoring it as an error of *rotation* according to the often-used scoring systems. Slope, in other words, is considered to be present if *any* slant may be detected at all. The hypothesis to be considered for this deviation is as follows: An upward slope (Figure 13.1) suggests that the subject tends to express or act-out his or her impulses; a downward slope (Figure 13.2) suggests some degree of depressed affect or a tendency to inhibit the impulses or drives that are experienced. Interpretively, of course, the greater the amount of slope that is seen in the figure that has been drawn, the more is the importance that should be assigned to what the deviation appears to be expressing.

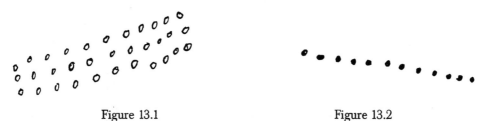

Figure 13.1　　　　　　　　　　　　　　　　　Figure 13.2

At times, slope will characterize only one part of a design. Here the interpretation will depend on when the slope takes place during the drawing of the design. If the slope is seen to occur first, and then is corrected (Figure 13.3), the hypothesis is that the subject tends to show the respective characteristic (depressiveness if slant is downward; impulsiveness or acting-out if slant is upward), but then regains control. If the slope does not occur initially, but occurs subsequently during the drawing of the design (Figure 13.4), the opposite interpretation is considered, i.e., the individual may be one whose initial reaction in a situation tends to be appropriate, but who quickly is overtaken by a depressive sense (downward slant) or by the tendency to act-out (upward slant).

Figure 13.3　　　　　　　　　　　　　　　　　Figure 13.4

Special Considerations for Unusual Features

The reader is reminded that attempts to reproduce the Bender-Gestalt designs may result in drawings that show unusual features or details that have not been discussed in this book, but that will nevertheless be recognized as causing the designs that are reproduced to appear noticeably different from the actual stimulus figures. At times, in fact, they may result in design drawings that appear to be remarkably disparate from the stimulus figures used as models. Many of these features are difficult to categorize into specific groups because of their very uniqueness and peculiarity and because they may be produced by individuals whose ego-functions are so seriously impaired that they often are clinically diagnosed on the basis of their aberrant behavior alone and without psychological testing with the Bender-Gestalt having been done.

On those occasions when an individual has not been diagnostically classified with a clinical syndrome (American Psychiatric Association, 1994), but is tested for other reasons, it sometimes does happen that drawing details considered to be signs of potentially severe emotional disturbance will be found in the Bender-Gestalt record. Children who are seen in school settings, having been referred for what appear to be academic or learning problems, may sometimes represent an instance of this circumstance.

In the author's experience, for example, there have been primary grade children who were suspected by their teachers of being intellectually retarded or of having a learning disorder and who were consequently referred in order to have that impression confirmed. When examined, however, it was found that the suspected "learning problems" were actually the side effects of serious psychopathology, for example, a pervasive developmental disorder. In such instances, the Bender-Gestalt records that were obtained frequently contained features such as open points of the hexagon, runovers at line junctures, breaks in lines, and peculiar elaborations.

Of the other drawing features that are difficult to categorize, perhaps the most apt term to describe them is *strange* or *odd*. This strangeness is sometimes in the form of a "feathery" quality that may be noted in the way the lines are drawn. Sometimes it is the presence of extra lines in the drawing that bisect or seem to cut off portions of the design. Or there may be elaborations of the design, not only in terms of extra lines, for example, but in the addition of features that turn the abstract design into a representational drawing that may or may not in itself be bizarre but, given the nature of the directions that are administered to the test subject, would certainly be considered a prominent deviation from expectation.

Verbal and Nonverbal Behavior

Those who approach clinical work from the perspective of projective psychology (Abt & Bellak, 1950) may regularly observe the tell tale signs of parallel communication that can be noted in the counseling client, the test subject, or people in general. Such communications occur, as Jung (1966) points out in his discussion of dreams, because the person unconsciously provides more information than is being asked for. In other words, while a respondent may *voluntarily* answer a question or comply with a direction, e.g., to draw something, he or she will *simultaneously and involuntarily* express inner conditions that may exist, such as impulses, emotions, or preoccupations, without recognizing that such additional communication is taking place. Projection occurs, then, because the expression of the additional information bypasses the person's defenses and the censorship that might otherwise be implemented in order to inhibit such self-disclosures.

With a facility that is quite remarkable, and through processes such as verbal and nonverbal condensation and symbolization, the unconscious consistently will provide a more complete and realistic picture of the private world of the individual than can be assessed through an exclusively quantitative analysis. It should be understood, of course, that unconscious communications are manifested in many areas of life experience, and not solely within the confines of the testing situation. In the more general contexts, however, they are not likely to be recognized for what they actually are. For those readers who would like to have the process of unconscious communication illustrated in the case of other psychological assessment methods, e.g., the Draw-A-Person, the Lowenfeld Mosaic Test, and the Rorschach, examples are to be found in Hammer (1981), Perticone and Tembeckjian (1987), and Phillips and Smith, (1953), respectively.

Chapter 5

SYMBOLISM AND THE BENDER-GESTALT DESIGNS

PRELIMINARY CONSIDERATIONS

The issue of whether or not specific meanings can be attributed to the stimulus figures of the Bender-Gestalt test has been controversial over the years. The outcomes of studies, using techniques such as the semantic differential, generally have been interpreted as being nonsupportive of the hypothesis of symbolic significance. However, as pointed out by Tolor and Schulberg (1963), many methodological problems can be found in the research addressing this issue.

In a subsequent review, Tolor and Brannigan (1980) again caution against too quick a decision to dismiss the possibility of symbolic meanings for the Bender designs. In doing so, they mention a number of justifications for their view, one of which appears to the present writer to be of major relevance and that is certainly consistent with the psychodynamic perspective that underlies the concepts and techniques offered in this book: They refer specifically to the notion that in order to test projective hypotheses, it may be necessary that activation of drives or conflict occurs in the research subjects or that the subjects are selected with consideration given to the personality conflicts or drive levels they are known to possess. Such conditions, of course, represent the precise circumstance that can be expected to exist in the actual clinical situation.

For example, when a client is motivated to seek counseling or psychotherapy or is undergoing a personality assessment, it is likely to be precisely because of the arousal of such conflict, that may or may not be consciously recognized, or because of the problematic effects of drive states that are being experienced. It is the author's view that when such conditions indeed do exist in the individual, it can be expected that *their presence will be expressed projectively* and, therefore,

41

that signs of their presence will be available for the clinician to discover.

INTUITIVE APPROACHES TO SYMBOLISM

When one has had extensive experience with a given diagnostic task, whether it be a mechanic pinpointing the source of car trouble, a physician searching for the cause of physiological disturbance, or a psychological examiner interpreting a test subject's responses, it is often the case that an accurate judgment is made concerning the meaning of an observed event or behavior even though the observer does not immediately know how the interpretive conclusion was reached. In some cases, this presumably occurs because the ideational processes leading to the insight have occurred below the observer's threshold of conscious awareness, although they subsequently may be deduced consciously. Excellent examples of this occurring in the clinical context are detailed by Reik (1956) in his book, *Listening with the Third Ear.*

In other instances, what is often referred to as *clinical insight* appears to be the result of what may be true intuition, i.e., a cognitively perceived outcome of the subjective and nonrational psychological process that has been described by Jung (1971) in his discussion of the *psychological functions.* When intuition occurs, the insight does not appear to be the logical outcome of the observer's linear thinking or reasoning.[1]   Many of the present readers who are clinicians involved in the practice of counseling, psychotherapy, or personality assessment probably can recall not only having experienced such an intuition but also finding that the intuition's accuracy was actually supported by subsequent events that unfolded in the therapy or assessment process.

The extent to which a clinician should attend to meanings or insights of the type alluded to above is likely to be hotly debated. Nevertheless, the position being taken in the present discussion is that intuition, although difficult to account for in an empirical manner, indeed may occur. Obviously, intuitively derived insights are subjective by nature. As such, they can and should be differentiated from conclusions and interpretations that are based on the results of controlled experimental studies. The fact that clinical intuitions are subjectively derived, however, does not necessarily mean that they are invalid. Indeed, they may be found to be not only valid, but to be extremely helpful in leading both the therapist and the client to the consideration of hypotheses that might otherwise be overlooked. Obviously, when a clinician does experience an intuition, it should be recognized for what it is and then subjected to corroboration from a variety of sources. A psychological examiner, for example, might check for the extent to which the clinical insight is consistent with conclusions derived from projective signs or quantitative scores obtained from other aspects of the same test, from data derived from other tests, from case history information, from self-report, and from other appropriate sources.

THE SYMBOLIC PULL OF THE STIMULUS FIGURES

In discussing the possible symbolic meanings that each of the Bender-Gestalt stimulus figures may hold for the test subject, it first seems wise to emphasize that interpretive hypotheses are not facts, but frames of reference from which facts, in the form of observations made of the subject's test behavior, can be given potential meanings. It goes without saying that these meanings, or psychological interpretations, must be subjected to rigorous clinical validation or confirmation in actual life functioning before being accepted as valid and put to practical therapeutic use.

In the presentation that follows, the Bender-Gestalt designs will be described one-at-a-time, and the particular dimensional and spatial features that are felt to have projective importance will be noted. Next, a general hypothesis will be given for the symbolic pull of each specific design. The types of unusual features that often are found in a subject's drawing of the design will then be described, and the psychological interpretations that are believed to be relevant will be presented.

Design A

The first stimulus to be presented to the subject, Design A, consists of two separate elements that make delicate contact with one another, i.e., they touch, but barely so. One figure is round, the other is angular. Although of differing shape, the figures give the appearance of being approximately the same size.

Hypothesis for Design A

Design A represents how the relationship with one's mother is experienced. Alternative, but less preferred interpretations, are that Design A symbolizes heterosexual relationships or interpersonal relationships in general.

Subjectively, this stimulus appears to have the quality of *twoness,* to coin a term. That is, although the circle and the square are each distinct shapes, they seem to constitute a pair. Because they touch each other, they appear to share a relationship.

The circle, which typically is drawn first, will be assumed to represent the mother or female figure. How the point of contact between the square and the circle is treated, therefore, is particularly important as a focus for symbolic expression.

When workover is present at the point of contact, the test subject may be projecting his or her experience of tension in the relationship. In Figure 14, the reworking of the circumference of the circle at the point where the square touches it seems to suggest that a barrier is felt to exist between the parties, as if the person represented by the circle is armored so as to be impenetrable, i.e., emotionally inaccessible.

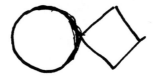

Figure 14

There are many other drawing details suggestive of the likelihood that the test subject may be experiencing relationship difficulties with the mother figure or a significant other. Relative size of the respective elements is one such feature. In Figure 15.1, the circle is seen to be considerably larger than the square. This suggests that the mother, female figure, or other significant person is perceived as being dominant in the relationship with the test subject. When the square is drawn larger than the circle, as shown in Figure 15.2, the opposite hypothesis is considered, i.e., the mother or other significant person is likely to be seen as being the submissive or less dominant member in the relationship.

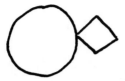

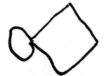

Figure 15.1   Figure 15.2

Another feature that may occur in the records of subjects having such interpersonal difficulties is the flattening that is sometimes seen in the drawing of the square element of Design A. This flattening may result in an elongation of the square in either the vertical or the horizontal direction (Figures 16.1 and 16.2). When this occurs, the hypothesis to be considered is that in order to maintain a relationship with the mother or significant other, the test subject must alter some aspect of his or her own nature or behavior, that is, inhibit or change some tendency that might otherwise be expressed. Such individuals typically feel considerable pressure to meet the needs and expectations of others and are fearful of the consequences of not doing so.

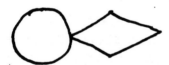

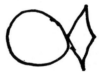

Figure 16.1   Figure 16.2

A variation of this is the flattening or elongation of only one part of the square. In Figure 17.1, the left half of the square is elongated as if it must be "stretched" in order to make contact with the circle. This may indicate that the test subject experiences great reluctance when faced with the possibility of interacting with the mother figure or her counterpart. Presumably, the subject functions more adequately until that interaction is imminent, as suggested by the fact that the portion of the square farthest from the circle is much more faithfully reproduced. When the half of the square making contact with the circle is accurately drawn, and the elongation or "stretching" occurs instead in the portion of the square that is farthest from the circle (Figure 17.2), the hypothesis is that the test subject is initially very reluctant to face, or interact with, the mother figure, but eventually mobilizes ego-resources or otherwise adjusts sufficiently so that when the interpersonal contact finally does occur, he or she is able to function in a well-integrated manner.

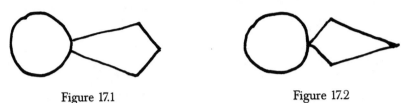

Figure 17.1   Figure 17.2

Interpersonal conflict or difficulty may also be hypothesized to exist when there is inaccuracy in the placement of the two elements of Design A. This may be expressed in the failure of the circle and the square to make actual contact with each other (Figure 18.1), in the square penetrating the circumference of the circle (Figure 18.2), or in the corner of the square that contacts the circle being open (Figure 18.3).

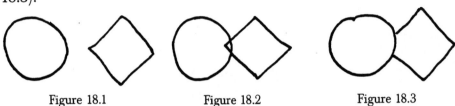

Figure 18.1   Figure 18.2   Figure 18.3

Failure of the two design elements to make contact with each other suggests emotional distance as will be dramatically illustrated by the anecdote that follows: A young adult female being seen in a counseling context was administered the Bender-Gestalt Test. Her completed record revealed one inaccuracy—Design A was drawn with a one-half inch space between the circle and the square. When all of the stimulus figures had been reproduced, she was again shown the card bearing Design A and asked if it looked the same as what she had drawn. Recognizing the error immediately, and answering in the negative, she then was given a new piece of paper and asked to draw it correctly by using the design on the stimulus card as a model. She redrew the design, but once more did so leaving a one-half inch space between the circle and the square. Questioned again, she acknowledged that she had made the same error, but that she did not mean to do so. She was once again requested to make an accurate reproduction, and once again made the drawing with the same error. At this point, she appeared perplexed and asked if she might try again. She did so another three times, but in each instance repeated the error, her reaction to this appearing to be one of shock and dismay. Since the testing in this case was being done for the purpose of guiding the counseling in which she was engaged, a decision was made to confront the client with the clinical implication of her repeated error. Consequently, the statement was made to her, "It seems that you have a huge difficulty in relating to your mom," to which she responded with a high degree of emotion, "God, yes! But how did you know?"

Penetration of the circle by the square is strongly suggestive of hostile feelings toward the mother figure or significant other and in some cases may imply that underlying sexual issues are involved. On the other hand, when the corner that touches the square is open, the hypothesis is that there is an oral-dependent aspect to the subject's relationship experience. In this latter instance, the greater the opening at the corner, the more prominent is the dependency need that is hypothesized to exist in the test subject's personality pattern.

Design 1

Design 1 consists of a row of twelve dots that are usually seen as having been placed equidistant from each other. In actual fact, the majority of the dots are placed in pairs.

Hypothesis for Design 1

The hypothesis for Design 1 is that it reflects the nature of the test subject's affective and behavioral tendencies when functioning in an individual interpersonal situation, i.e., when relating only to one person.

As was seen to be the case with Design A, each of the hypotheses discussed previously under the heading of *Specific Design Features* can be stated with more explicit contextual implications when the symbolic pull of the specific design is kept in mind. The importance of considering the combinations of unusual features that may be present in the drawing of a design will be elaborated more fully in later sections of this book.

With respect to Design 1, circles substituted for dots (Figure 19.1) suggests that the test subject's manner of relating to others will be characterized by immaturity when in a one-to-one situation, perhaps to a greater extent than would be so when in a group circumstance. (This latter qualification may be corroborated by the manner in which

Design 2 is drawn, as will be explained later.) Similarly, if the the dots are drawn as dashes (Figure 19.2), impulsivity also may be predicted when the interpersonal context is an individual one.   Sometimes many, or even all, of the dashes will have been so rapidly drawn that they will actually be seen to resemble the letter Z when they are close- ly scrutinized by the examiner (Figure 19.3). In the author's experi- ence, "zee-ing" is a very strong indicator that impulsivity is so great a trait in the test subject that his or her behavior, when observed in actu- al life situations, will often be dramatically inappropriate.

Figure 19.1	Figure 19.2	Figure 19.3

A slope in an upward direction (Figure 20.1) strengthens the hypothesis that acting-out is likely when the situation involves only one other person. Slope that is in a downward direction (Figure 20.2) may indicate that unhappiness will be the characteristic mood experi- enced in such an interpersonal situation

Figure 20.1	Figure 20.2

Projective features such as those mentioned above, or others not yet mentioned, may be combined in the reproduction of a single Bender-Gestalt design. It will be necessary, therefore, for the examin- er to consider these features as they interact with one another in order to derive meaningful and integrated hypotheses concerning the test subject's personality functioning. To illustrate, the reproduction of Design 1, as shown in Figure 21, would be interpreted as suggesting an individual who, when in a one-to-one context, may be expected to present a satisfactory adjustment pattern initially. It is further antici- pated, however, that he or she will rapidly lose some degree of emo- tional control and begin to behave immaturely and in an impulsively expressive fashion, perhaps when some familiarity with the other per- son has been established. This behavioral sequence is suggested by the observation that the first dots that are drawn, those at the left, are reasonably well-reproduced, but deterioration of accuracy begins to occur early during the execution of the drawing. Soon, it is noted, the dots become enlarged and then are drawn as circles, suggesting that the test subject's immature proclivities are beginning to be manifested. A further departure from accuracy is found in the upward slope that begins by the time the drawing is half completed and becomes pronounced by the time it has been finished. An upward slope, it will be recalled, is hypothesized to be indicative of the tendency to act-out.

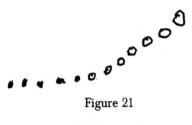

Figure 21

Design 2

This design is usually perceived of as eleven parallel columns, each column containing three small circles arranged so that it slants from left at the top to right at the bottom. On rare occasions, it may be seen instead as consisting of three parallel rows of circles that are placed horizontally, with the same amount of space between each of the rows, and with each succeeding row being slightly indented.

Hypothesis for Design 2

As was the case with the preceding design, this Bender-Gestalt stimulus figure represents the way in which the test subject is likely to behave interpersonally, but this time when the social situation involves relating within a group context rather than on an individual basis. In addition, it is hypothesized that Design 2 reflects the test subject's response to group relationships in general rather than to functioning in any particular social group within the life space, e.g., the family.

Slope again may be interpreted as being suggestive of either a depressive or an acting-out tendency depending on the direction of the slant, downward or upward, respectively (Figures 22.1 and 22.2), while dashes substituted for circles (Figure 23) again points to impulsivity and to a proclivity for acting-out.

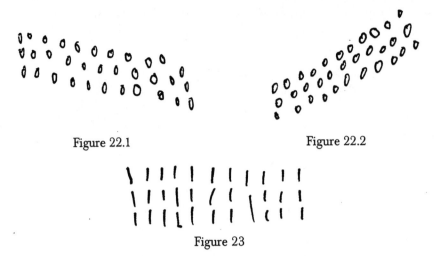

Figure 22.1   Figure 22.2

Figure 23

Another feature of interest is the shortening of the horizontal dimension of the overall design that occurs when several of the columns of dots have been omitted in the drawing (Figure 24). This latter feature is interpreted as indicating the test subject's preference for limiting group involvement to gatherings that are relatively small. By extension, this suggests that discomfort may be experienced when the test-subject is required to take part in large group situations.

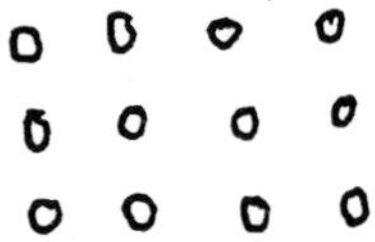

Figure 24

In the interpretation of any of these projective indicators for Design 2, the position taken by the author is that the behavioral tendencies that are suggested refer to occasions in which the test subject happens to be involved in a group situation. It follows, then, that of particular interest to the projective examiner will be the relationship of the hypotheses generated in response to the subject's reproduction of Design 1 to those generated in connection with the manner in which Design 2 is drawn. It will often be found, for instance, that tendencies such as acting-out or depression may be hypothesized for the test subject when he or she is in a group situation, but not when the social circumstance is limited to a one-to-one interaction. The converse may also be the case. Clinically, the detection of this differential tendency will be particularly helpful in determining whether a particular individual may be helped more by increasing or decreasing the degree of involvement in one type of interpersonal context in favor of the other, for example, group versus individual. It is possible, of course, to find that the behavioral tendencies that are hypothesized may be predicted to occur in both individual and group social contexts or in neither. In the former instance, the specific design features, e.g., slope, substitutions, etc., will probably be found to be present in both the Design 1 and the Design 2 drawings. In the latter case, the projective features will probably be absent in both.

As should be obvious by this point in the discussion of the interpretation of the stimulus pull of the designs, any combination of unusual features may appear in the test subject's drawings. These may include not only the full appearance of one of the variations already discussed, but the occurrence of that feature only in part or only to a slight degree within the design that is drawn, i.e., not pronounced enough to constitute a scoreable error. However, the point was made before and is being reiterated now that *any* deviation in the drawing by a test subject, who is not seen as developmentally disabled or organically impaired, should be scrutinized for its projective implications, particularly in the case of older children, adolescents, and adults.

Design 3

This stimulus figure also consists of dots arranged in a symmetrical fashion. It begins with a single dot that is succeeded to the right by a shallow angle comprised of three dots, that in turn is succeeded by an angle of equal degree that is made up of five dots, followed by an another equivalent angle consisting of seven dots. The single dot, that is to the left, establishes the left terminus for the horizontal line formed by the dot that is at the point of convergence for each angle. The design is commonly, but not always, thought of as pointing from left to right.

Hypothesis for Design 3

It is hypothesized that this design symbolizes the ego-drive of the test-subject. As such it may be considered an indicator of assertiveness, motivation, or the tendency toward self-expression. When circles are substituted for dots in this design (Figure 25.1), it may be hypothesized that the test subject's drives or motivations are probably immature in either their focus, their expression, or both. Dashes substituted for dots (Figure 25.2), suggests that drives are likely to be expressed in an impulsive fashion. As discussed earlier, when the attempt to draw dashes is recklessly fast, the "dashes" may appear to be in the form of the letter *Z* (Figure 25.3). This should be considered a prominent indication of impulsivity that is extreme enough to result in interpersonal problems. As should be anticipated, these interpretations will take on added significance when slope in an upward direction is also noted in the drawing, since the acting-out of any impulsive tendencies will be considered to be an increased likelihood.

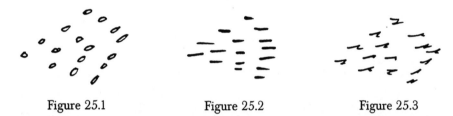

Figure 25.1   Figure 25.2   Figure 25.3

Distortions in shape may result when the attempt is made to reproduce Design 3. Whatever forms such errors of distortion may take, they generally will reflect the tendency of the test subject to experience problems when dealing with, or attempting to satisfy, various psychological needs. In this connection, the manner in which the test subject draws the succeeding angles of this design is especially worthy of the examiner's attention. The hypothesis is that the more acute the angles, the more likely is the test subject to express his or her drives in an assertive, and possibly hostile, manner. Figure 26.1 illustrates moderately pointed angles in the drawing of Design 3. By contrast, the angles in Figure 26.2 will be seen to be acute.

Figure 26.1   Figure 26.2

Sometimes it will be observed, however, that some or all of the angles lack pointedness. In Figure 27.1, for instance, all angles are blunted, suggesting that a failure to express oneself assertively is a consistent trait. In Figure 27.2, only the final angle (at the right end of the design) is sharp, while the preceding "angles" are blunted or rounded. In this case, the interpretation is that in various circumstances the individual is likely to be hesitant to act assertively, but finally will be able to do so even though such assertion does not come easily.

Figure 27.1   Figure 27.2

In contrast, some individuals have the inner experience of needs or drives that they would like to satisfy, but when the opportunity to do so presents itself, these inclinations are likely to be inhibited or even totally suppressed. This interpretation would be made when considering a drawing such as that shown in Figure 27.3, where the first and second angles are reasonably sharp, but the final "angle" is definitely blunted. Figure 27.4 shows a drawing of Design 3 in which no angles occur at all. Here, the interpretation would be one of an individual who may be characterologically lacking in assertiveness and who, as a result, is likely to be seen by others as rather conforming and possibly inclined toward passivity.

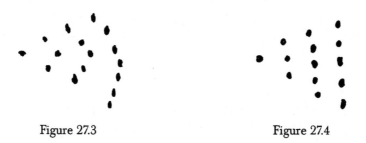

Figure 27.3   Figure 27.4

Other projective features whose interpretive hypotheses will interact with those discussed above are slope and the substitution of circles or dashes for dots. An upward slant in the design drawn by the subject strengthens the hypothesis that drives will be acted-out. If circles have been substituted for dots, the expression of ego-drive is likely to be seen by others as immature or regressive in nature. This is also strongly indicated if dashes are substituted for dots and an upward slope is present in the drawing.

Design 4

Design 4 consists once again of a line drawing comprised of two separate elements that touch each other at only one point. The element at the left is an open square, i.e., the top side of the "square" is missing. The element at the right is a bell-shaped (curved) line, the midpoint of which makes contact with the lower right hand corner of the open square.

Hypothesis for Design 4

The symbolic pull of this figure appears to be similar to that of Design A in that it is hypothesized to elicit associations pertaining to the test subject's relationship with the mother figure. Also, as was the case with Design A, the alternative, but less preferred hypothesis, is that it symbolizes the nature of a specific heterosexual relationship or possibly heterosexual relationships in general.

The presence of workover is again an important feature for the examiner to identify, since the treatment of the connection of the two elements in this figure is likely to reflect how the test subject feels or thinks about his or her relationship with the mother figure, or other significant person, and what means are emphasized in the adjustment to that relationship. At times the workover will occur at the lower right corner of the square, but often the whole right side will be heavily reworked as shown in Figure 28.1. When this happens, not only is the experience of tension suggested, but it can be hypothesized that the cause of the strain between the the two individuals is attributed by the test subject to the mother or other significant person.

On other occasions, reworking of the lines at the point of contact will be present in the curvilinear element and not in the square (Figure 28.2). This can be interpreted as suggesting that it is the test subject from whom the resistance and subsequent tension are perceived to stem.

Should the workover be present in both the square and the curved line at the juncture point, it is hypothesized that the antagonism will be perceived by the subject as being attributable to the attitudes or actions of both parties. An example of this may be seen in Figure 28.3.

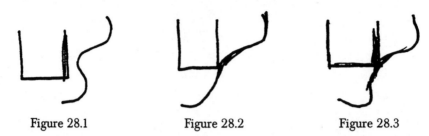

| Figure 28.1 | Figure 28.2 | Figure 28.3 |

In Design 4, as was discussed in connection with Design A, there is sometimes a deficiency in the integration of the two elements that comprise the total stimulus figure. As shown in Figure 29.1, this may take the form of the failure of the square and the curve to make contact. When a gap does result from the failure to integrate these two parts correctly, it is believed to be a projective indicator of the inability of the test subject and the mother figure to establish or maintain emotional contact with one another. Sometimes such a failure to integrate the two design elements will occur in combination with workover in either the square, the curve, or both (Figure 29.2). When this does happen, the interpersonal difficulty can be hypothesized to involve not only a sense of alienation in the respective individuals, but it is also probable that considerable tension is felt by the individuals in connection with their troubled relationship.

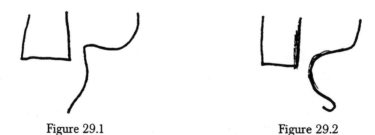

Figure 29.1   Figure 29.2

The examiner should also be alert to another interesting variation in the presentation of these features in the design reproduction. This is the highly symbolic gesture of connecting the separated elements with a single, and often lightly drawn, line (Figure 29.3). Such a projective communication may be interpreted as reflecting either the highly tenuous effort by the test subject to connect with, i.e., relate to, the other person or the attempt to create a facade of doing so. The former alternative implies that there may be a willingness to maintain the interpersonal tie, even if it is an unsatisfactory one. The latter hypothesis suggests that some purpose is being served by creating the appearance of an adequate or normal relationship, but that any external manifestations of the interpersonal bond will be found to be superficial when investigated more thoroughly.

The failure to achieve a correct integration of the two elements of Design 4 may also be seen when they overlap. When this occurs, the curve (usually drawn second), will appear to be penetrated by the lower left corner of the square (Figure 29.4). The interpretation of such penetration is that hostility is experienced by one or both of the parties concerning their relationship with each other and that confrontation between them can be expected. This view is given further projective support if an upward slope is present in the drawing.

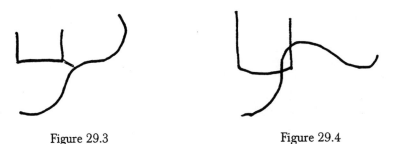

Figure 29.3   Figure 29.4

An additional feature that, in the author's experience, has been found to be clinically revealing is the rotation that may occur when Design 4 is attempted. The reference here, of course, is to the test subject whose history, performance record, and results from other testing serve to contraindicate the likelihood of any organic involvement. Further, the rotation that is alluded to is that which occurs in the open square portion of the stimulus figure and is one of approximately 180 degrees. A simultaneous rotation usually is not present in the curvilinear portion of the design (Figure 30).

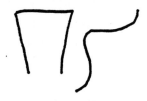

Figure 30

Such rotations make it appear as if the square is in an "upside down" position. This appears to be of great projective importance to some subjects because the open square, when in its orientation as shown on the stimulus card, may appear as a container that is capable of holding something. This is an allusion to its potential as an unconscious symbol for the womb and may be why Design 4 seems to elicit unconscious associations pertaining to the mother figure. When an open "container" is inverted, of course, its contents will be dropped or spilled out. Taken together, these thoughts lead to the hypothesis that the inversion of the open square may well imply a profound sense of maternal rejection in the test subject.

An example showing how a maternal rejection experience can be indicated by the rotation of the open square of this Bender-Gestalt figure is illustrated by the case of a nine-year-old boy who was undergoing a full test battery in connection with an educational placement decision that was in the offing. The youngster was examined on two separate occasions with a space of one week between the first and the second test session. The Bender-Gestalt Test was administered during session one, at which time Design 4 was drawn as shown in Figure 31.1. It was decided, however, to administer the test again during session two for purposes of personality assessment because of the rather sullen appearance of the test subject when he arrived for the second visit. This time, Design 4 was drawn by the youngster as depicted in Figure 31.2 where, it readily may be seen, the open square has been rotated approximately 180 degrees. Following the test session, the matter was investigated through an interview in which it was revealed that during the intervening week a disruptive argument had taken place between the test subject and another family member. The mother acknowledged that her reaction to the altercation was one of intense anger toward the boy and a feeling of not wanting to be around him for a while, a sentiment that was certainly detected by the youngster.

Recognition that a dynamic interaction of this kind, one that even may typify the relationship, has occurred or is presently occurring can be of great help to the psychotherapist or counselor. It is often the case that such circumstances are not readily acknowledged by either of the parties who are involved, the result being that an interpersonal difficulty of great significance may not be dealt with in a timely fashion in the treatment process.

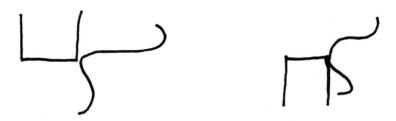

Figure 31.1   Figure 31.2

Of the many other types of unusual features that may be present in the drawing of Design 4, two more will be discussed here. These pertain to distortions in the shape of the curvilinear element and to the complete closure of the open square.

The first of these, i.e., distortion of shape, is seen either in a flattening of the curve at the point of contact with the square (Figure 32.1) or a compression of the curve such that it appears to be elongated in its height (Figure 32.2).

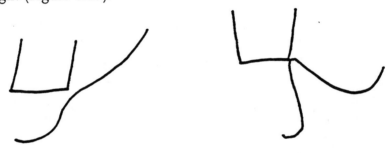

Figure 32.1   Figure 32.2

When flattening occurs in the curved element, the hypothesis is that the affect that is experienced in connection with the mother figure is one of sadness or depression. The greater the flattening, the more pronounced the depressed affect is presumed to be. By contrast, compression of the curve so that it is elongated and appears to be "stretching" in order to contact the open square suggests that the test subject is able to relate to the mother or significant other, but is hesitant, or finds it difficult, to do so.

The term *relate*, as it is used in this hypothesis, refers to both the subjective inner experience associated with the interpersonal relationship, for example feelings, thoughts, and attitudes, or the external behavioral manifestations of relating to the significant person that may be observed directly by others.

Complete closure of the open square element of Design 4 (Figure 33) also suggests relationship difficulties. Here, it may be hypothesized that the mother figure or significant other is seen as emotionally inaccessible. The consequence of this for the test subject may be the experience of affect-deprivation and a sense of hopelessness about the possibility of a deep emotional relationship with that parent or significant person.

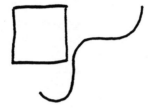

Figure 33

Design 5

Design 5 is created entirely of dots that are arranged more or less in the shape of an incomplete circle or arc, with a straight extension consisting of dots extending from off-center right at the top of the arc. The arc is made up of nineteen dots; the extension consists of seven dots.

Hypothesis for Design 5

It is hypothesized that this design elicits projections of the test subject's perception of his or her familial or home environment. In the case of adults, it may pertain to the emotional ambiance that was experienced during childhood or it may refer to the home as it is experienced in the present. It also may reflect conscious or unconscious memories of both.

In this design, circles being substituted for dots (Figure 34.1) may be seen frequently in the records of children, adolescents, and adults. From the perspective of personality assessment, this feature is hypothesized to be an indication that feelings about, or responses to, the home environment have been immature in character. In the case of the older test-subject, this may imply regression, especially if any previous testing with the Bender-Gestalt Test has not resulted in this reproduction error. If testing over time demonstrates consistency in the test subject's use of circles instead of dots in drawing this design, however, it is probably fixation that is being indicated. Such a differential assessment, of course, can be of use in determining the psychotherapeutic approach that can best be utilized for a given client.

As shown in Figure 34.2, dashes are sometimes used instead of dots when reproduction of this design is attempted. The hypothesis for this occurrence is that hostility is experienced in connection with the home. Difficulty in inhibiting impulses may also occur in that environment.

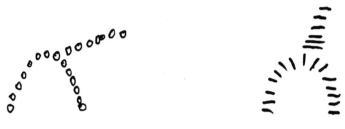

Figure 34.1   Figure 34.2

Slope also is often seen in drawings of Design 5. As with other designs, the slant may be in an upward or a downward direction (Figures 35.1 and 35.2, respectively). When the slant is upward, a potential for acting on impulses is indicated, an interpretation that takes on added significance if slope occurs in combination with the substitution of either circles or dashes for dots. When slanting downward characterizes the reproduction, the affect experienced in connection with the home is hypothesized to be dysphoric or gloomy.

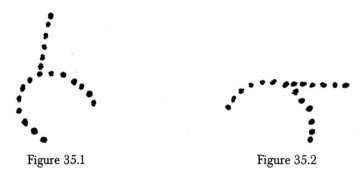

Figure 35.1   Figure 35.2

Design 6

Design 6 consists of a horizontally placed wavy line that is intersected at a slant by another wavy line. The curves of both lines are sinusoidal, but those of the horizontal line are wider than the curves of the intersecting line.

Hypothesis for Design 6

This Bender-Gestalt design is hypothesized to be reflective of the affective state of the test subject. As such it is seen to be sensitive to transient emotions as well as moods.

One of the more commonly encountered projective indicators in drawings of Design 6 appears to be that of changes in the amplitude of the curves, particularly in the horizontal line. When the height is noticeably reduced (a special instance of flattening) the hypothesis is that the test subject's affective state is one of sadness, depression, or melancholy. An example of this is given in Figure 36.1. As in the other types of flattening previously discussed, the degree of depression will be suggested by the extent of the flattening. Greater flattening, in other words, indicates a greater degree of depression.

When the height of the curves has been increased beyond that depicted on the stimulus card (Figure 36.2), a high degree of emotionality is anticipated in the client, either subjectively experienced or expressed outwardly. The degree of amplitude must also be considered. If the height reached by the curves is pronounced, hysterical acting-out is a possibility. This hypothesis is supported if the lines have been drawn very rapidly, i.e., impulsively, and the behavioral tendency is even more to be expected if fewer or extra curves have been drawn in the respective lines.

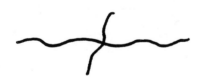

Figure 36.1   Figure 36.2

The presence of slope in the drawing of this design is again interpreted as indicating either a depressive quality or a tendency to express affect outwardly. When slope does occur, it is usually in the design as a whole. An upward slant to the design is suggestive of acting-out (Figure 37.1). When the slant is directed downward, (Figure 37.2), unhappiness or a similar depressive condition is indicated. As should be expected, slope will increase the significance of any amplitude or flattening that characterizes the curves of either line.

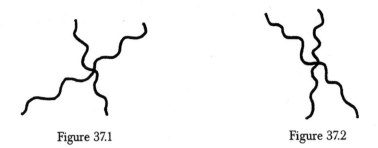

<table>
<tr><td>Figure 37.1</td><td>Figure 37.2</td></tr>
</table>

Design 7

This Bender-Gestalt figure is made up of two elongated hexagons that overlap. They are placed so that the narrow dimension of each is in the vertical plane, with the left hexagon leaning to the right. The point at which they intersect is at the top portion of each hexagon. The intersection itself is not total. That is, although one hexagon overlaps the other, it does so only partially.

Hypothesis for Design 7

Design 7 is hypothesized to indicate the nature of the test subject's relationship with the father. The presence of so many angles is believed to facilitate unconscious associations with a masculine figure, with males in general, or with the concept of maleness.

This Bender-Gestalt design appears to be one of the more difficult to reproduce, and problems in drawing it are not uncommon in test subjects below the age of ten and even below the age of eleven. While the complexity of Design 7 certainly appears to be directly related to maturational variables, it is also interesting to speculate on the extent to which its symbolic significance contributes to its challenge for the drawer.

With regard to personality assessment, this design often appears to be a trigger for anxiety, hostility, and even confusion in the test subject. Indications of such affective or cognitive experiences often may be inferred from the actions and demeanor of the individual when attempting to reproduce it. The examiner may sometimes notice, for example, indications of autonomic changes (respiration, flushing, etc.), spontaneous comments, and behavioral manifestations such as fidgeting, unnecessary erasing (often at the point of intersection), and the like.

In clinical work over the years, the author has found that this design is, for the test-subject, similar to Design A and Design 4 in that it also seems to convey the quality of "twoness," i.e., of being a pair. In the case of Design 7, it is presumed that the symbolism of pairing involves the subjective association of a prominent male figure, probably the father or a father representation.

Workover frequently is seen at the point where the two hexagons overlap. The projective hypothesis to be entertained when this is observed is the likelihood that the relationship with the father or prominent male is characterized by tension or conflict. At times the workover will be limited to the lines of one hexagon, and at times it will be found in the other. In either case, the interpretation is that the difficulty in the relationship is perceived by the test subject as stemming primarily from one of the two individuals involved (Figures 38.1 and 38.2). When the workover occurs in both the right and the left hexagon (Figure 38.3), it is hypothesized that both parties are perceived to be contributing to the defensive armoring and tension that is experienced between them.

    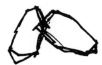

Figure 38.1   Figure 38.2   Figure 38.3

Integration errors occurring in Design 7 include those in which there is no overlap of the hexagons and those in which the overlap is exaggerated. As was noted in the discussions of the placement of the two elements in Design A and the two elements in Design 4, regardless of the type of error of integration that occurs, the projective implication is that a noteworthy relationship difficulty exists.

When the hexagons are drawn so that neither is in contact with the other, as shown in Figure 39.1, the hypothesis is that emotional distance is experienced in the relationship with the father figure. Whether the difficulty is felt to be the fault of one party or the other sometimes may be inferred from spontaneous comments made by the test subject or by responses given during the Free-Association and Selective-Association phases of the test. In addition, the degree to which the hexagons are separated from each other in the drawing may provide a clue to the magnitude of the interpersonal alienation or separation that is felt by the examinee.

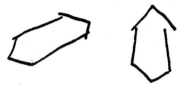

Figure 39.1

At times, while there may be no intersection of one hexagon and the other, there nevertheless is some contact made between these two elements. Figure 39.2, for instance, shows the right and left hexagons side by side in a more-or-less parallel manner. Here, it is hypothesized that there is a minimal emotional relationship with the father figure or, perhaps, the need to create the appearance of rapport or connection, albeit a superficial one. The fact that the hexagons are parallel and the same size suggests that the issue of psychological parity with the father or other male figure is of particular importance to the test subject.

Figure 39.2

At the other extreme of the integration errors is the exaggerated penetration of one hexagon by the other (Figure 39.3). This feature is hypothesized to indicate that very significant discord is experienced in the relationship with the father figure. Whether the affects and cognitions associated with the conflict are experienced primarily at an internal level or whether they are likely to be expressed externally in the psychosocial world, e.g., as open hostility or acting-out, may be inferred by other features present in the drawing. The presence of slope in one or both of the hexagons, workover of lines, and/or angles that are highly pointed or drawn with slashlike movements support the hypothesis that the conflict is openly expressed. Lines that are very lightly drawn or hexagons that are smaller than the models shown on the stimulus card suggest that feelings and thoughts about the father figure, although experienced by the test subject, are probably inhibited.

Figure 39.3

Design 8

This is the final Bender-Gestalt design to be administered to the test subject. It is most often seen as consisting of an elongated hexagon placed in a horizontal position. Within, and at its center, is a diamond that is slightly longer (top to bottom) than it is wide. It is also possible for this design to be seen as two horizontally placed hexagons that overlap at the point where the diamond is typically perceived.

Hypothesis for Design 8

The hypothesis that is proposed for Design 8 is that it facilitates a projection of the test subject's perception of the ego or the phenomenal-self (Combs & Snygg, 1959) in the life space. The diamond, largely because of its central place within the hexagon that contains it, is presumed to serve as an unconscious representation of the phenomenal-self. The surrounding line, in the form of a hexagon, represents the dimensional world in which that self operates.

Given the hypothesis stated for Design 8, its position as the final figure to be drawn appears to be psychologically most propitious. As a representation of how one sees himself or herself in the world context, the response to it will to some extent reflect or encompass all the personality characteristics, focuses of the test subject's attention, and dynamics that were considered in the discussion of the hypotheses associated with the preceding Bender-Gestalt designs combined, including:

1. The impact of one's relationship with each of the parental figures, and the symbolic representations of them in later life, e.g., authority figures, spouses, and any number of significant others.
2. The degree of comfort experienced in interpersonal relationships outside of the family, both individual and group.
3. The strength and regulation of ego-drives.
4. The influence of the familial environment on one's sense of personal security and comfort.

5. The nature of the emotions that are prominent in the individual's experiences and the manner in which the emotions are regulated or expressed.

In considering the test subject's reproduction of Design 8, it again will be important for the examiner to identify the unusual features that may be present in the drawing so that hypotheses may be generated concerning their implications for personality functioning. In addition, however, it may be very useful to assess the extent to which those hypotheses are consistent with, or disparate from, the ones derived from the examiner's analyses of Designs A through 7. Should a disparity exist, it may very well be an indication of particularly effective defenses having being employed by the test subject. In terms of Bender-Gestalt Test performance, this may be expressed as follows: When problematic personality characteristics and conflicts are revealed by the test subject through the projections occurring in the preceding design drawings, but no unusual features are noted in the rendition of Design 8, the hypothesis is that the individual is attempting to portray the facade of a conflict-free existence in the world about him or her. The opposite interpretation should be entertained when the preceding design drawings show few or no unusual features, but their presence is clearly discernible in the production of Design 8. That is, the individual manifests to self and others an awareness of disharmony or difficulty in coping with the world, but is denying the specific issues and dynamics that are behind such problems.

Disproportion in the comparative size of the hexagon and the diamond naturally may be in two directions: The hexagon may be large and the diamond small, or the hexagon may be small and the diamond large. When the diamond is drawn too small, it may be placed so that it touches the top, but not the bottom line of the hexagon (when the latter is drawn in the horizontal plane). A second possibility is that the diamond may touch the bottom, but not the top of the hexagon. The third possibility is that the diamond may appear to be "floating," i.e., touching neither the top nor the bottom line of the hexagon.

Smallness in the size of the diamond suggests feelings of personal inadequacy and inferiority. When an undersized diamond appears to be suspended from the top line of the hexagon (Design 40.1), it may be hypothesized that the individual tends toward fantasy, perhaps as a means of compensating for his or her imagined shortcomings. The placement of the diamond so that it contacts the bottom side of the hexagon (Figure 40.2) hints that the feelings of inadequacy are accompanied by marked dependency characteristics or behavioral manifestations. When the diamond, in its smallness, appears to be "floating" within the interior of the hexagon, i.e., there is no contact with any of the hexagon's sides, feelings of isolation and possible withdrawal tendencies are suggested (Figure 40.3)

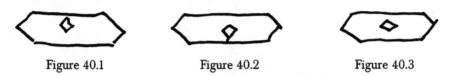

Figure 40.1   Figure 40.2   Figure 40.3

Disproportion in size of the respective elements of this design may also be noticed in drawings in which the size of the diamond has been exaggerated, or conversely, the hexagon has been made relatively too small. If either of these conditions obtains, it sometimes will result in the top or the bottom point of the diamond extending beyond the boundaries demarcated by the sides of the hexagon that are supposed to contain it. More often, however, the penetration will be found to occur at both ends of the diamond as shown in Figure 41.1. In the case of any of these alternatives, it is hypothesized that the test subject perceives the world to be very constrictive. In other words, the individual probably feels very pressured by what are seen as the demands and expectations of others. This typically translates into the belief that people wish to control him or her. Given such perceptions, the world is likely to be viewed as a hostile one that perhaps must be challenged if one is to be successful in meeting personal needs.

If workover is present in Design 8, it more commonly will be found in the drawing of the diamond rather than the hexagon. When this occurs in conjunction with the diamond being of exaggerated size (Figure 41.2), it may be hypothesized that not only does the individual experience pressure from the world about, but also that there is likely to be considerable tension and hostility felt concerning it.

Slope is another feature that frequently will occur in combination with the projective indicators mentioned above. In Figure 41.3, an upward slope will be noted in the hexagon in addition to both workover and exaggerated size of the diamond. Taken together, these drawing details indicate that the individual's response to the tension and the control issues that are being experienced internally will probably find outward expression. That is, interpersonal conflict is not expected to remain covert, but likely will be acted-out in the social context.

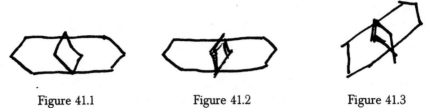

Figure 41.1   Figure 41.2   Figure 41.3

The final unusual features that will be discussed in connection with Bender-Gestalt Design 8 are gaps in angles, broken lines, and runover of lines in the drawing of the hexagon. All of these are considered to be particularly important occurrences because it is hypothesized that they sometimes may portend the weakening, or even the impending failure, of ego-defenses.

In attempting to reproduce Design 8, the test subject at times will leave a gap in the angles that make up the pointed ends of the hexagon (Figure 42.1). Such gaps may be indicative of a potential loss of impulse control. The larger the gaps, the more the seriousness that should be attached to the potential clinical implications of this feature. There also may be gaps (Figure 42.2) at the juncture of the lines making up the more shallow angles of the hexagon. These may be present instead of, or in addition to, gaps that occur at the pointed ends of the design as described above. Similarly, the hexagon, and more rarely the diamond, may be drawn with lines showing many breaks (Figure 42.3). Breaks in the lines are also suggestive of weakened ego-integrity.

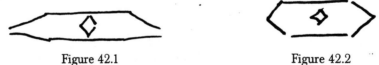

Figure 42.1   Figure 42.2

At times runover will be noted at the point where lines converge to form an angle (Figure 42.4). When any of these features is present, the hypothesis is that ego-integrity has been weakened and that the emotional adjustment of the individual may be tenuous. Usually there is an accompanying awareness in the individual of personal vulnerability to both inner and outer forces that are perceived to be beyond his or her control. Such individuals may be expected to feel very apprehensive as they attempt to cope with their day-to-day activities because they are fearful that "something bad" may happen.

| Figure 42.3 | Figure 42.4 |

The features described above may appear in combination with some of the other signs that already have been discussed. As is invariably the case, the examiner must be aware of such combinations of projective features that may appear in the designs drawn by the test subject and then consider how the hypotheses associated with each of the projective signs may support, mitigate, or amplify one another.

INTERPRETING THE RECORD: A CASE EXAMPLE

In the following material, a Bender-Gestalt record will be interpreted for the purpose of illustrating the approach to hypothesis-building as described under *The Symbolic Pull of the Stimulus Figures.* In this simulation, only the test subject's sex, age-range, and response time will be indicated. No information will be provided concerning case history, presenting problems, reason for referral, or results of other testing, all of which certainly would be highly important considerations in an actual clinical case being followed in practice. Nor will observations be given concerning the test subject's behavior and manner during testing. The intentions here are only to demonstrate what projective features the examiner might identify in the design drawings themselves and to summarize the interpretations that might be considered and for which supportive evidence would then be sought.

The Bender-Gestalt record which is presented in Figure 43 will be found to contain a number of features having projective significance. These may be noted in the appearance of the protocol as a whole as well as in the drawings of the individual designs. For this reason, some preliminary interpretive comments will be offered that pertain to the test subject's protocol in general.

Sex of Subject:	Male
Age of Subject:	Middle Adolescence
Total Response Time:	One Minute, Twenty-three seconds

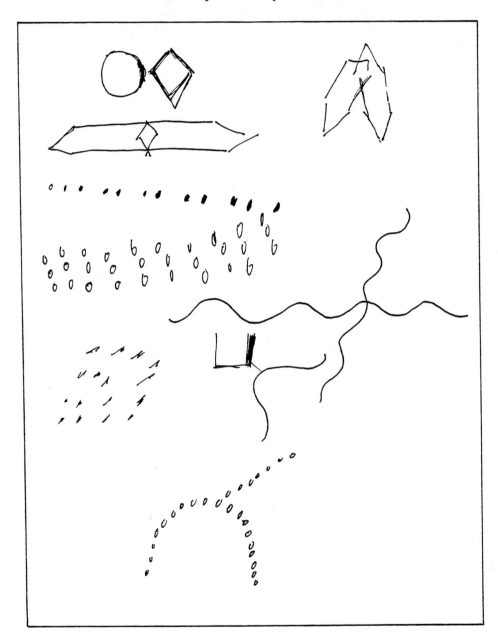

Figure 43

General Observations

The drawings rendered by this subject capture the basic gestalts of the separate designs, and although some features are present which might approach the criteria for the scoring of errors in some quantitative systems, e.g., slope in Design 3; circles substituted for dots in Design 5, this does not appear to be a function of a neurological deficit. Instead, impulsivity and excessive tension are likely to account for such "error" tendencies in the perceptual-motor responses These personality characteristics are suggested, respectively, by the very brief period of time required to complete the nine drawings and the heavy pencil pressure that was necessary in order to produce such dark and heavy lines.

Mental astuteness and accuracy of perception are suggested by the correct number of dots in Designs 1 and 3, rows and columns in Design 2, and sinusoidal curves in Design 6.

Also of general interest is the test subject's utilization of space. The fact that most of the paper has been used for the task suggests that the individual is unlikely to withdraw from social interaction. Indeed, it seems probable that his presence in the interpersonal environment will be a prominent one as is suggested by his tendency to draw the designs so boldly and, in a number of instances, to make them relatively large.

The arrangement of the designs on the paper is disorderly, but not chaotically so. Placement may be seen to be logical and sequential initially, but it becomes somewhat disorganized as Design 4 is reached, with Designs 6, 7, and 8 appearing to be inserted without apparent concern for orderly sequence. This pattern, in combination with the test subject's brief response time, indicates that he may approach interpersonal and other situations methodically and with satisfactory emotional control at first, but has the propensity to become impatient and soon will act impulsively instead.

Interpretation of the Individual Designs

Design A

The initial drawing is placed logically and is of appropriate size, suggesting the ability to perceive the environment accurately and to plan ahead. There is considerable workover present, however, with the lines of the square being heavily reinforced. These features suggest that the test subject experiences a high degree of tension and discomfort, probably concerning his relationship with his mother and possibly with females in general. That he is probably uncertain how he should present himself to such figures is indicated by the first attempt at drawing the square.

It will be noted that the lines making up the bottom-most corner of the square were initially drawn too long so that the resulting figure was noticeably distorted. Interestingly, in making the correction, there has been no attempt to remove the incorrect lines so that the final image appears to be superimposed on the former. The hypotheses that follow observation of these features are that the test subject's judgment becomes impaired when experiencing interpersonal stress and that more than one aspect of his personality may be apparent to the observer in an interpersonal situation, i.e., the other person may see through the persona that the test subject is attempting to present.

Design 1

This design is also placed logically and consists of the correct number of dots, suggesting that attention to detail remains good. Perceptual accuracy and some compulsivity are indicated by the grouping of the dots in pairs, a feature that also hints to the likelihood of at least average, and probably above-average, intelligence. The slight, but apparent, downward slope of the row suggests the presence of some dysphoria or a depressive tendency that possibly has resulted from an unconscious activation of intrapsychic conflict that may have been stimulated by the symbolic pull of Design A. The depressive quality may become apparent when the individual finds himself in the relative intimacy of an individual social interaction.

The first dot, it will be observed, is drawn as a circle. This suggests that a tendency to regress, i.e., to feel or behave immaturely, is likely to be the initial response in a one-to-one interpersonal situation. That efforts to control this tendency will probably be through the use of intellectual defenses is indicated by the test subject's return to the drawing of dots and the arranging of them in pairs, the latter feature being a typically obsessive-compulsive pattern. Such ego-operations are only partially successful, however, and the individual experiences a building up of inner tension and frustration as reflected in the successive increase in the size and boldness of the dots as they are drawn.

Design 2

Placement of Design 2 continues to follow an orderly sequence, and again shows accurate attention to details in that the correct number of rows and columns of circles are drawn. There is a decided slope in an upward direction, however, that indicates that the test subject possesses a propensity to act more impulsively when he finds himself in a group social context rather than he does when in an individual social situation. The waviness that is seen in the rows of circles points to an increase in emotional instability when in such a group setting. This feature, in combination with the upward slope of the drawing, suggests that the emotions that are experienced are likely to be expressed outwardly.

Design 3

Although the sequential placement continues, the test subject's rendering of Design 3 provides mounting evidence of emotional disturbance. This suggests that the self-assertiveness and ego-drive that tend to be symbolized by this design are likely to be expressed in a hostile manner and without reflection. These hypotheses derive from the following observations: The arrow-like figure shows a pronounced upward slope, suggesting an acting-out tendency; the angle at the right, the last one drawn, is quite acute, the pointedness indicating an incisive hostility; dashes are soon substituted for dots, with "zee-ing" also occurring in the final angle. Taken together, these features indicate a distinctly impulsive personality style that is characterized by low frustration tolerance and a high potential for the acting-out of hostility.

Design 4

For the first time, a shift in placement of the drawings is noticed, with Design 4 being positioned more centrally on the sheet of paper. That this shift has been made despite sufficient space being available to continue the previous top-to-bottom pattern of design placement suggests that it may carry a personal significance that is being unconsciously projected. This leads to the hypothesis, in other words, that whatever is being symbolized to the test subject by Design 4 does have a specific and central meaning in his life, i.e., it pertains to core issues that are relevant to his personality dynamics and development. As was also suggested by the treatment of Design A, these issues are presumed to involve the individual's relationship with his mother or mother representations.

In addition to its placement, two other peculiarities can be seen in the drawing. These are the marked workover which occurs on the side of the open square which is closest to the curvilinear element, and the failure of the subject to integrate correctly the separate elements that make up this design.

Projectively, the presence of marked workover at the precise location where it occurs may reflect the test subject's perception of a mother figure that is emotionally inaccessible to him. It is as if a wall or barrier has been erected between them that makes a warm and meaningful connection all but impossible. One might further deduce that this has deep-seated psychosexual and dependency implications, a hypothesis that might be well worth exploring in psychotherapy. In any event, the presence of conflict centering on the maternal relationship is strongly indicated.

Scrutiny of the drawing will also reveal that a short and faint line has been drawn in the space separating the curve and the square. This is interpreted as reflecting the highly tenuous nature of the relationship he wishes to portray himself as having with the mother figure. Alternatively, it may constitute the symbolic expression of a very feeble attempt to satisfy his frustrated dependency need.

Design 5

In the drawing of Design 5, which is hypothesized to symbolize the experience of the familial environment, placement is similar to that of the previous design, but lower. The most noteworthy feature, however, is the substitution of circles for dots. This is seen as being indicative of regression and is hypothesized to indicate an immature attitude of the individual toward his home and an immature pattern of responding to family members.

Design 6

The drawing of this design to the right and above that of Design 4 results in the most pronounced deviation in the placement sequence thus far. The reproduction is fairly good, with the height of the sinu-soidal curves being only slightly elevated. Since Design 6 is presumed to reflect the manner in which the test subject experiences affect, the hypothesis is that the individual appears able to manage his emotions consistently and in a generally modulated fashion despite the impul-sivity that is believed to characterize him, and even though it has been hypothesized that he experiences major relationship conflicts with sig-nificant others.

The appearance of emotional balance suggested by the initial observations of the manner in which this design has been rendered, however, may be largely an expression of persona, i.e., the test sub-ject's need to create the impression that he is adequately controlled emotionally rather than emotionally overreactive. This is suggested by the exaggerated size of the design which implies that despite the general accuracy of the intersecting wavy lines, emotional experience is probably quite prominent for him. The hypothesis that there is a potential for more intense affective experience is also supported by the fact that the placement of this design is so close to that of Design 4 that the latter is almost encompassed by it. The drawing of Design 4, it will be recalled, was already interpreted as reflecting a major adjustment issue.

Design 7

This design, drawn in the upper right corner of the paper, again shows that the test subject grasps the essential relationship of the sep-arate elements to each other and is able to integrate them quite well. This is interpreted as indicating a more satisfactory perception of the father figure than was hypothesized for the mother. Nevertheless, the light workover which is present indicates that some tension is felt in the connection with the father, while the broken line in the right hexa-gon may be an indication that psychological trauma has been experi-enced by father or son. The failure to close angles, particularly notice-able in the left hexagon, suggests that loss of impulse control may be likely to occur in the relationship between the two.

Design 8

The drawing of the final Bender-Gestalt design is inserted in the space between the drawings of Designs A and 1. Although its gestalt remains essentially intact, the hexagon is disproportionately long and somewhat compressed from top to bottom. Projectively, this suggests that the test subject feels considerable environmental pressure and perceives the life space to be confining and constrictive. Because the top and bottom points of the diamond extend beyond the upper and lower sides of the hexagon, it is hypothesized that the individual's response to the pressure he feels is to push beyond the limits that are set for him.

SUMMARY AND CONCLUSIONS

Projective analysis of this Bender-Gestalt record suggests that the test subject is an adolescent, probably of above-average intelligence, who is experiencing significant adjustment difficulties in terms of both intrapsychic processes and social relations. He appears to be highly impulsive, hostile, very tense, and prone to acting-out. This appears to be a characterological pattern which likely is rooted in faulty parent-child relationships of long-standing duration. At a deeper level of experience, unresolved dependency issues and psychosexual conflict are likely to be prominent in his dynamics. This person should be referred for a full psychological evaluation. Both individual psychotherapy and family participation appear to be indicated.

ENDNOTES

1. Elements of the insight or intuition, however, may sometimes be subsequently categorized and therefore understood in a manner that makes the insight appear to be more consistent with what is familiarly defined as *reasoning* (Jung, 1971, p. 454).

Chapter 6

INTERPRETING THE
VERBAL ASSOCIATIONS

SPONTANEOUS AND
EXAMINER–ELICITED VERBALIZATIONS

It seems reasonably safe to assume that the Bender-Gestalt Test traditionally has been thought of as a perceptual-motor technique in which verbal involvement is limited either to the examiner's instructions to the test subject or to the test subject's questions about them. Nevertheless, some workers (Clawson, 1962; Yonda, 1984) have found it useful to elicit oral responses to the test subject as well.

Certainly, it has always been possible for the examinee to make spontaneous verbal comments before, during, or after the completion of the task. Undoubtedly, most psychological examiners, as a consequence of their training as observers of behavior, have listened for, and been sensitive to, such utterances, particularly when what has been spoken pertains to feelings, abilities, or past experiences that have obvious relevance to the personality of the individual. Comments such as, "I'm not good at drawing," or, "That didn't come out right, but it's the best I can do," are easily recognized as being self-evaluative in nature, for instance, and that as such they may constitute clues to the speaker's self-concept or manner of coping with real or imagined criticism. Similarly, traits such as dependency and deference to authority are suggested by questions about how to proceed, e.g., "Does it have to be the same size," or, "Should I put in all the circles?"

In the same way, issues of trust as well as attitudes toward the examiner, and presumably other authority figures, are implied by verbalizations such as, "What are you going to do with this stuff when I'm finished?" or as one school-age youngster was heard to complain, "Every time I'm asked to do one of these things, something bad happens to me." This latter remark, of course, points to previous evaluation efforts that have resulted in specific and distasteful consequences for the test subject.

The implications of comments or questions of the type alluded to above should be fairly transparent to any experienced psychological examiner. There are *other* types of verbalizations that are made by a test subject, however, that may be equally or even more revealing, but are commonly excluded from many examiners' consideration. These are the seemingly innocuous words, phrases, and sentences that are uttered and which, on the face of it, *seem* to be meaningless or otherwise irrelevant to the personality assessment process.

The present author wishes to emphasize the view, however, that tremendously useful insights are often derived from an analysis of such wordage. For this reason, the psychological examiner is again strongly encouraged to proceed on the assumption that not just some, but *each and every verbal communication uttered by the subject is psychologically meaningful* and, furthermore, that *it is likely that different messages are being presented simultaneously, although at different levels of awareness.* Consequently, *every* utterance by the test subject should be examined not only in terms of its manifest message, but with due regard for the covert communication that may be imbedded in, or symbolically connoted by, the literal words that have been spoken.

It is also most important to consider the context in which the verbalization occurs. This requires the examiner to identify what the subject was doing immediately before, as well as during, the time the remark was made. To illustrate, an adult male test subject is heard to comment, "Maybe I should turn this around," when he is first presented with Design A for reproduction. He is then observed to rotate the stimulus card counterclockwise by ninety degrees so that the square element is at the top and the circle is at the bottom. At a surface level, the remark (or the action taken) appears to be an expression of his thought that the design might be easier to reproduce if the stimulus card is placed in a vertical, rather than the horizontal, position.

In this instance, one hypothesis is that what has been revealed by the utterance might be the test subject's awareness of a need to compensate for some difficulty in spatial orientation. At a psychodynamic level, however, a collateral hypothesis is that the test subject is communicating a conscious or unconscious drive to assume or maintain dominance in a relationship, probably with the mother figure or some other significant person. In other words, he feels the need to be "on top" in the relationship. The fact that the test subject's verbalization is spoken in the context of his response to Design A, rather than another design, is the reason that the hypothesis has been given this particular interpersonal focus.

Another example of the importance of what at first glance may appear to be spontaneous wordage that has no relevance to personality assessment, but in fact is actually both meaningful and highly relevant, is the following: While attempting to intersect the two hexagons in her drawing of Design 7, a young adult female test subject is heard to utter, seemingly to herself, "That's never going to come out right." The manifest meaning of this remark seems to be an indication that the drawer anticipates that her attempt at reproducing the design will probably fall short, as far as accuracy is concerned. While this may be a true *conscious* intent of the communication, the examiner may also hypothesize that the test subject is *unconsciously* and *simultaneously* expressing her awareness of an underlying unresolved conflict with the father figure, or another person who probably is perceived as possessing stature or authority. This hypothesis is derived because the examiner presumes the possibility exists that the communication contains a *parallel* thought or meaning, and therefore is prepared to recognize the multiple messages that are being communicated. By bearing in mind the symbolic pull of Design 7, the subject's words, "That's never going to come out right," can be thought of as a reference to a relationship with a specific person in her life rather than as a remark which simply and exclusively concerns the relationship between the abstract geometric shapes that are being drawn.

The principle being stressed here is that verbalizations, including those that appear to be spontaneous chitchat, often will be found, on examination, to contain multiple messages. Furthermore, such multiple messages are communicated by individuals, both in and out of the examination experience, to a far greater extent than is usually realized. Simply having the awareness that parallel communications do indeed take place, however, may in itself result in an increase in the examiner's sensitivity to its occurrence in the clinical situation with the result that valuable clinical interpretations may be made concerning them.

THE FREE-ASSOCIATION PHASE

It will be remembered that in this phase of the expanded Bender-Gestalt administration, the test subject is asked to provide associations to the stimulus figures by reporting what each seems to resemble or what each "makes you think of." The examiner records the responses and all ancillary remarks and behaviors, observes if the stimulus card is turned or if it is maintained in the position in which it was first presented, and notes the amount of time elapsed prior to the first association being communicated.

In interpreting this phase of the test, all the principles which have previously been discussed concerning a test subject's spontaneously emitted verbalizations are also applicable. The examiner should be alert, for instance, to:

1. Connotations of the words being used.
2. Use of the *double entendre* or punning words.
3. Changes in auditory volume, pitch, or verbal fluency.
4. Autonomic indicators such as blushing.
5. Other relevant behaviors, verbal or nonverbal, that are noted.

The reason that such observations should be made and evaluated is that they commonly are the telltale accompaniments of ideas, attitudes, and feeling states that exist internally but are not volitionally disclosed because either the test subject is loathe to admit them to others or because he or she is unconscious of their existence. They may be thought of, in other words, as "flags" that signal to the examiner the presence of dynamics that are clinically relevant to the individual's personality functioning.

Because the associations in this phase of testing are made to stimuli for which the symbolic significance is already anticipated by the examiner, an additional level of meaning of the test subject's responses often may be deduced, and hypotheses about personality functioning consequently may be stated more specifically than would otherwise be the case. For example, if a test subject's association to Design 4 is, "It looks like a nose pressed against a block of ice," the examiner might reasonably hypothesize that the response may reflect a feeling of emotional coldness that is experienced by the individual. If it is also remembered that the association is given specifically to a design for which the symbolic pull is already hypothesized to center about perceptions of one's relationship with the mother figure, the hypothesis becomes much more focussed and essentially points to an area to be investigated more deeply through further testing with methods, for example, such as the *Thematic Apperception Test,*[1] and explored through interview or in the psychotherapy sessions which may follow the assessment that is being undertaken.

In developing the hypothesis illustrated in the above simulation, it may be helpful to review the observations and analyses that lead the projective examiner to the specific psychological interpretation. These can be divided into the following process segments:

1. The response that is given includes the concepts *nose, pressed, block of ice.*
2. *Nose* may be a phallic symbol, suggesting that it is a male who is the doer of the action, in this case the test subject himself.
3. *Pressed* implies that energy is being expended, suggesting the existence of an active drive, need, or motivation to achieve a goal.
4. That the energy has "pressed" the nose against the ice, a substance that is by nature both cold and hard, suggests that the effort is not resulting in an experience of emotional satisfaction, i.e., warmth, but one that is its opposite. (A person who is described as "cold" is typically seen as rejecting or hard to relate to emotionally.)
5. Design 4 is tentatively assumed by the examiner to stimulate unconscious perceptions of one's mother. Here, the open square is a classic uterine symbol, and it is at this point that the "nose" is seen to be "pressed."
6. The tentative conclusion follows that it is feelings about the mother, or possibly other persons who have become the psychological representation of the mother, that will be found to be a major source of affectional frustration for the individual or, perhaps, an unresolved Oedipal conflict.

Needless to say, this is an example of the projective analysis of a specific association by one test subject to one specific design. It should be understood that associations to the various designs can be expected to vary greatly among those who are administered this phase of the expanded approach to the Bender-Gestalt. It is, in fact, precisely such variability that makes the process of projective analysis possible. As has been succinctly stated by Frank (1948):

The essential feature of a projective technique is that it evokes from the subject what is, in various ways, expressive of his private world and personality process. The projective technique gives the subject the opportunity to invest situations with his own meaning, to impose upon them his own values and significance, especially affective significance.(p. 47).

In order to demonstrate further the interpretive outcomes of projective assessment in the Free-Association Phase of Bender-Gestalt testing, several examples of associations of the type that might be made to each of the nine designs by different test subjects will be presented. Inquiry that would be made by the examiner will be indicated by a Q in parentheses (Q). An Initial Reaction Time (IRT) will be given for each of the associations presented. Suggested projective interpretations will then be stated. Some brief commentary may be offered, but the reader is encouraged to make his or her own interpretive deductions according to the format that was illustrated above in order to deduce how the projective conclusions were reached. When considering hypotheses about the associations that are obtained from the test subject, it will be important, of course, to bear in mind the symbolic pull of the individual designs.

Design A

Association (Adult Female, Single)   IRT: 08"

"When I first saw it, it looked like objects you're looking down on . . . like a square peg and a round peg. It's an aerial view."

Projective Interpretation

Perception of a faulty relationship with a significant other, possibly a mother representation, or of feeling out of place in some social situation. Incompatibility is implied. "Aerial view" suggests a disdainful attitude toward the relationship or situation and a wish to distance oneself from it.

•••••••••••

Association (Adult Male, Single)   IRT: 13 "

"It looks like a sign . . . Road signs . . . like a . . . stop sign and a caution sign."

Projective Interpretation

Doubt about a relationship is prominent in the test subject's mind. Fears that it will be dangerous to proceed too quickly in the relationship and that perhaps he should stop his involvement altogether.

•••••••••••

Association (Adult Female, Married)   IRT: 10"

"Maybe opposites that are together." (Q) "Maybe a man and a woman."

Projective Interpretation

Marital difficulty. Perception of incompatibility that may or may not be consciously admitted.

•••••••••••

Association (Middle Adolescent Female)   IRT: 03"

A sperm trying to penetrate an egg. That's all I can think of."

Projective Interpretation

Sexual preoccupation. Possible pressure to engage in sex, but conflicted about this. Obsessive tendency.

•••••••••••

Design 1

Association (Older Adult Male)   IRT: 09"

"Ants." (Q) "Little ants marching in a straight line."

Projective Interpretation

Feelings of inferiority. Pressure to conform to expectations and standards of others. Deference to authority. May lack spontaneity.

•••••••••••

Association (Young Adult Male)   IRT: 12"

"They look like the dots you would find in the books that they use to teach kids. It looks like they need to be connected. Something is missing."

Projective Interpretation

Regressive tendency or immaturity.   Feelings of alienation. Unsatisfied desire for a meaningful one-to-one relationship.

•••••••••••

Association (Older Adolescent Male)   IRT: 36"

"My mind is a blank . . . I don't know . . . I don't know . . .It's like seeing bars from the top, I suppose. Like in a jail cell."

Projective Interpretation

Feeling trapped.   Sense of being punished and restricted. Repression and denial are likely to be commonly used defense mechanisms.

•••••••••••

Association (Older Adolescent Female)   IRT: 08"

"That one looks exactly like the dotted line down the middle of the road . . . so you can know where you're going."

Projective Interpretation

Insecurity feelings. Hesitance to act independently. Conformity to the expectation of the other person when in a one-to-one relationship. Perfectionistic tendency.

•••••••••••

Design 2

Association (Adult Female)   IRT: 30"

"I don't like this one very much because there are so many circles and it's hard to get them in alignment . . . I suppose it looks like an audience."

Projective Interpretation

Experiences discomfort and is insecure when in group situations. Feels as if under scrutiny of others. May feel pressure to perform. Wishes to influence the perceptions or behavior of others, but doubts competence to do so.

•••••••••••

Association (Older Adolescent Male) IRT: 11"

"Eyes. There are many eyes . . . in the dark. They're watching you.

Projective Interpretation

Paranoid sensitivity. Environment perceived as potentially dangerous.

•••••••••••

Association (Young Adult Female) IRT: 06"

"That looks like a bunch of people in some kind of group . . .

Like they're having a good time . . . and maybe dancing. They seem to be swaying in synchronization with each other."

Projective Interpretation

Social interest. Probably extraverted. Wishes to be a part of, and to participate in, group activity. Absence of social anxiety.

•••••••••••

Association (Adult Female) IRT: 45"

"Ooh . . . This is strange . . . It reminds me of viewing something . . . almost in a perspective . . . like . . . rows and rows of tombstones. I didn't want to say . . . I didn't want to say that."

Projective Interpretation

Morbidity. Has need to understand life experiences associated with death or loss, but attempts to avoid thinking about. Ideas intrude, nevertheless. Resorts to defense mechanism of denial to escape unpleasant feelings and thoughts.

•••••••••••

Design 3

Association (Female Elementary School Child) IRT: 05"

"Oh boy! This looks like a pretty Christmas tree, but we have to hold it this way." [Rotates stimulus card 90 degrees to the right]. "Do you like it, too?"

Projective Interpretation

Age-appropriate response. Is probably a spontaneous child. Appears assertive and able to test limits, but still needs reassurance from adult that her behavior is acceptable. Respect for authority.

•••••••••••

Association (Young Adult Female)   IRT: 04"

"That one I see as a process . . . a definite growing process. It keeps forming out."

Projective Interpretation

Drive for personal development and self-discovery. Appears self-motivated and self-aware. Ability to form abstract concepts.

•••••••••••

Association (Adult Male Combat Veteran)   IRT: 03"

"Oh God! A frightening experience. Army stripes."

Projective Interpretation

Traumatization. Possible posttraumatic stress

•••••••••••

Association (Young Adult Male)   IRT: 14"

"It really looks like the head of a spear, but it could be going in either direction. I'm not sure which. One end is very sharp and the other end isn't so sharp. The whole thing seems to be disintegrating."

Projective Interpretation

Pronounced ambivalence about self-assertion, the form it should take, and the direction to be followed. When confronted with important decisions, may experience major drop in ego-strength.

•••••••••••

Design 4

Association (Adult Female)   IRT: 27"

"Hmmm." [Sighs] "It's a conflict. It's something that's soft and something that's hard . . . striking each other." (Q) "The box- like thing is what's hard. Empty and hard."

Projective Interpretation

Interpersonal strife and frustration. Perceives a significant other, possibly the mother figure, as intransigent and unable to provide either nurturance or support.

•••••••••••

Association (Adult Male)   IRT: 16"

[Shakes head] "These are things that . . . I don't like the way they fit together." (Q) [Shakes head] "Nothing really . . . They don't work well together, as I see it."

Projective Interpretation

Interpersonal difficulty with a significant other, possibly the mother figure. Perceives incompatibility and little hope. Appears to see problem only from his own perspective. Poor prognosis for improvement.

•••••••••••

Association (Female Elementary School Child)   IRT: 08"

I think that somebody is getting hit over the head with something.

Projective Interpretation

Feelings of vulnerability, possibly in relation to mother figure. Anticipates hostility from significant other.

•••••••••••

Association (Adult Male, Single)   IRT: 14"

"This looks like a breast. A woman's breast. And I never picked up on the open-ended square . . . . . . Except the point is going right where the nipple would be."

Projective Interpretation

Immature sexual preoccupation. Possible psychosexual fixation and unresolved Oedipal issues. Hostility in connection with mother figure, a female, or females in general.

•••••••••••

Design 5

Association *(Male Elementary School Child)*   IRT: 04"

"It's an igloo and it's being attacked by an enemy space invader. Kaboom!"

Projective Interpretation

Experience of the home environment as rejecting or unsatisfying. Hostile impulses directed toward the home. Use of fantasy as a defense.

Association (Early Adolescent Female)   IRT: 02"

"That looks like an exploding planet. The flare is coming out. Lots of heat energy."

Projective Interpretation

Accumulated tension. Awareness of emerging sexuality. May involve experiences or fantasies within the familial environment. Phallic preoccupation. Possible abuse.

•••••••••••

Association (Young Adult Female)   IRT: 06"

"Oh no! It could be a collar with a leash . . . maybe for a dog. It's a dog's life!"

Projective Interpretation

Perceptions of being controlled or restricted by others. Feels unhappy, but is probably resigned to it.

•••••••••••

Association (Adult Female, Single)   IRT: 11"

"The first thing that comes to mind is protection. There is something inside the semicircle . . . and . . . it's being protected from invasion."

Projective Interpretation

Feelings of vulnerability. May look to the home for safety. Alternatively, may be a counterphobic reaction to fears stemming from the home environment. Experiences sexual anxiety. Fear of penetration.

•••••••••••

Design 6

Association (Young Adult Female)   IRT: 15"

"This is two people's paths that have crossed. One is going faster than the other. Maybe too fast."

•••••••••••

Projective Interpretation

Awareness of difference in motivations, probably in a specific relationship. Uncertainty and apprehension about the consequences.

•••••••••••

Association (Adult Male, Single)   IRT: 05"

"I think that what we have here is two curvy roads that finally meet at the top of a mountain."

Projective Interpretation

Experiences emotional fluctuations. Use of the pronoun we implies an interpersonal relationship, and it may be that this is what is perceived to be difficult. Appears to be optimistic about final outcome. Tends to be persistent.

•••••••••••

Association (Adult Female)   IRT: 02"

"Ugh! That's that damn roller coaster. Up-down. Up-Down. I don't know why on earth they call it an amusement park!"

Projective Interpretation

Pronounced mood swings. Possible cyclothymia. Possible biologic involvement. Emotional frustration.

•••••••••••

Association (Adult Male)   IRT: 05"

"Well, this could be a stream flowing through the forest. Another one is flowing into it. A good fishing stream. Right here is where they connect."

•••••••••••

Projective Interpretation

Emotional balance. Easygoing temperament. Recreational interest. Is possibly reflecting an interpersonal relationship about which he feels emotionally satisfied.

•••••••••••

Design 7

Association (Adult Female, Married)   IRT: 17"

"It reminds me of crystals. They are . . . lying against each other . . . Going in opposite directions. Lying next to each other, but there is no communication. They're hard."

Projective Interpretation

Pronounced frustration in relationship with a male, probably the husband, or possibly the father figure.   Marital difficulty likely. Experiences deprivation of affectional needs. Inability to negotiate the problem, and perhaps even to discuss it . Pessimistic about outcome.

•••••••••••

Association (Older Adolescent Male)   IRT: 11"

"What comes to mind right away is . . . an automobile accident. Two cars that have run headlong into each other."

Projective Interpretation

Hostility and interpersonal conflict, probably with the father or other authority figures. Tendency toward opposition rather than submission.

•••••••••••

Association (Male Elementary School Child)   IRT: 07"

"Chunks of chalk . . . like what you try to write with. They got all broken up."

Projective Interpretation

Feelings of inadequacy, possibly related to school work. Possible learning problem.

•••••••••••

Association (Young Adult Female)   IRT: 12"

"They remind me of mice. Squashed mice. Like they've been stepped on and thrown on a rubbish heap."

Projective Interpretation

Inferiority feelings. May have experienced abuse. Possibly fearful of father or men in general.

•••••••••••

Design 8

Association (Adult Male)   IRT: 40"

[Looks at back of card] "This is hard . . . I'm not sure what to do with it . . ." [Rotates card and returns to original position] "I think . . .

I suppose it could be an eye. The center could be the pupil. Yes, that's what it could be. It's not perfect, though." (Q) "I guess it could be looking at you . . . or watching you."

Projective Interpretation

Feels insecure in the life space. Sense of being scrutinized by others. Probably self-evaluative and conscious of own performance. Recognizes faults in authority figures, but is nevertheless sensitive to their expectations or opinions. Obsessive tendencies. Tends to see environment as judgmental or hostile. Paranoid sensitivity.

•••••••••••••

Association (Adult Female, Married)   IRT: 17"

"Dear me. This could be like you are looking down on a wedding band. This is the design on it. It has a design instead of a diamond . . . to make it look valuable."

Projective Interpretation

Marital dissatisfaction. Probably regrets having married. May expend energy in attempt to maintain appearance of a satisfactory relationship.

•••••••••••••

Association (Young Adult Male)   IRT: 09"

"It looks like total disintegration. There is a smaller one . . . and it exploded. Watch out! The smaller one exploded . . . or is going to."

Projective Interpretation

Feeling burdened by environmental pressure. Anticipates imminent loss of control. Possible danger to self or others.

•••••••••••••

Association (Young Adult Female)   IRT: 05"

"Indecision." (Q) "There is a central theme, but there are two ways of looking at it. See, it's pointing in opposite directions, but exactly the same on both sides."

Projective Interpretation

Is experiencing major ambivalence, possibly about directions in life. Options appear equal so that conflict remains unresolved.

•••••••••••••

In considering the associations to the Bender-Gestalt designs and the projective hypotheses generated for them, it is necessary to be open to alternative interpretations that may be warranted by the data, but that may not have been entertained. For this reason, it is advocated that the examiner routinely ask himself or herself, following the development of any hypothesis about a verbal association, "What else might the words that have been spoken be communicating?"

It is also essential to be aware of the ways in which other observations about the test subject's performance (e.g., initial reaction times, hesitations in speech, etc.) or ancillary information about the subject (e.g., age, marital status, gender, etc.) will increase or decrease the relevance of an interpretation that is considered or even if an interpretation should be considered at all. The communication of developmentally simple verbal concepts for example, may not appear significant in the associations of a young child, but may be quite significant if given by an adult. Conversely, more sophisticated verbal concepts may not be considered noteworthy if obtained from an adult, but may appear very noteworthy if articulated by a young child.

THE SELECTIVE-ASSOCIATION PHASE

In this phase of the testing, the attempt is made to influence intentionally the direction of the test subject's associations to the stimulus figures. Instead of simply assuming that the Bender-Gestalt design being responded to has a symbolic meaning, e.g., mother, for Design 4, the word *mother* will be spoken by the examiner in order to indicate clearly that this is the image or perception to which the visual association is to be made.

While lengthy verbal comments occasionally may be made by a test subject when he or she is complying with the examiner's directions, it will be found that in most cases the verbalizations will be brief. In fact, in some instances, no words may be spoken at all, and the response only will be made nonverbally. The test subject, for example, may simply point to the specific design intended, or simply tap with a finger the card bearing the design. Whatever the mode of response, however, it is to be recorded or described exactly as it has occurred.

In the following discussion, the Selective-Association Phase of the administration will be demonstrated by providing examples of the stimulus words that might be delivered to a test subject by an examiner. Descriptions of the kind of verbal and/or nonverbal responses that could be made by the test subject will then be illustrated. When inquiry is felt to be important for the purpose of clarifying a response, it will be indicated by the letter Q in parentheses (Q).

In these examples, identification of the test subject will be limited to information such as age-range, gender, etc. To elicit each selective association, the examiner's directions to the test subject will have begun with words such as, "Which one do you like . . . ?" (most, least, etc.) or, "Which one makes you think most of . . . "(mother, father, etc.).

When all of the responses for one subject have been reported, a commentary will be offered concerning projective implications of the data. Once more, when considering the selective associations of the test subject, and how they are communicated, the reader should remain alert to the symbolic pull of the design to which the association is being made.

Example One: Adult Male, Unmarried

Like Most? : Points to Design 4. Strokes card with index finger.

Like Least? : Appears indecisive. Eventually taps Design 7 with middle finger.

Mother? : Points to Design 4. Smiles. Touches card with index finger.

Father? : Scrutinizes all the designs. Frowns. After sixty-two seconds says, "I have to reach for that one! I'd just as soon close my eyes and pick one . . . Nope. I can't get a clear association on that one no matter how hard I try. I haven't the foggiest idea."

Self? : Laughs softly. Points to Design 7. "The one I like the least." Shakes head from side-to-side.

In this example, there are several observations that are of interpretive importance. It is noted, for instance, that the first three responses are nonverbal. In selecting Design 4 as the one liked most, the test subject may be acknowledging a positive identification with his mother. The fact that he actually strokes the card suggests a tactile need which in turn may be a hint that there is an immature quality to the affectional relationship with the mother figure. This hypothesis is supported by the selection of Design 4 again, this time to designate the explicit association to the stimulus word, *mother.*

Designation of Design 7 as the one liked the least, however, indicates the possibility of an impaired relationship with the father. That there is conflict in connection with this relationship is also suggested by the apparent indecisiveness in dealing with this design. That the conflict probably involves strong feelings of hostility is indicated by the middle finger being used repetitively to identify Design 7 (the middle finger being the one that is commonly used to make a well-known gesture of derision or to communicate anger).

Further support for the hypothesis of a seriously strained relationship with his father is seen in the length of the test subject's initial reaction time when directly requested to associate to his father. Here, there is a change in that the response is not only verbal, but is surprisingly wordy. Despite the abundance of words, however, no design is designated. This, like the indecisiveness noted when asked which design was liked least, implies defensiveness and an attempt to avoid facing or admitting the problem. The avoidance is also connoted by the statement, "I'd just as soon close my eyes," words that suggest the defense mechanism of denial. The expressions, "I can't get a clear association . . . no matter how hard I try," and, "I haven't the foggiest idea," point to his confusion and inability to make sense of the problem, even should he attempt to do so.

The selection of Design 7 as the one reminding him of himself may at first seem unexpected. Theoretically, however, the identification that this response seems to suggest he makes with his father, especially in view of the immature dependency relationship he appears to have with his mother, may actually be a reflection of a long-standing psychosexual problem centering on unresolved Oedipal issues. Shaking the head, as if communicating, "No," may reflect both his confusion and his defense of denial in this regard.

Example Two: Older Adolescent Female

Like Most? :   Touches Design 3 with index finger. Pauses and then says, "No. Forget that." Touches Design 2 and says, "Better make it this one."

Like Least? :   Touches Design 8 with index finger. Eyes have become slightly moist.

Mother? :   Nods head as she touches Design 1 with index finger.

Father? :   Sighs. Points to Design 5.

Boyfriend? :   Moves card bearing Design 7 to the left.

Self? :   Touches Design 8 with index finger.

In this example, the test subject's initial response is a nonverbal one. She then designates Design 3 as the most liked, but changes her mind and chooses Design 2 instead. This behavioral sequence appears to be an expression of her wish to be assertive or to move toward a goal. Having symbolically communicated this, it is hypothesized that she then experiences conflict and feels the need to deny or inhibit her ego-drive. This is suggested by her saying, "No. Forget that." Her next utterance, "Better make it this one," which is spoken as she designates a different design, seems to suggest her surrender to a superego value that perhaps is not truly her own. From this point, it is observed that she is more inhibited in responding, as evidenced by her restricting herself to nonverbal communications. The replacement of her first choice with this particular design may point to her involvement in group social activities instead of expressing her individuality and may represent a compensation for not doing the latter.

By choosing Design 8 as the one liked least, the test subject may be indicating that dissatisfaction is being experienced concerning her life circumstances. That she is unhappy about her situation seems to be indicated by the hint of tearfulness which is occurring as she considers her response. Limiting herself to a nonverbal form of communication suggests both that she is inhibiting self-expression and that she tends to accept her situation passively, but painfully.

Design 1 is chosen as the design that reminds the test subject of her mother. There is no verbal indication given of her feelings about the relationship with this significant figure, but the nodding of her head, as if indicating the affirmative, may be a sign that she sees it positively, an interpretation which possibly may be supported by hypotheses formulated during Phases One and Two of the testing.

The test subject probably perceives the father to be the central power in the family constellation, as indicated by her selection of Design 5 when asked to associate to him. Given the hypothesis of self-inhibition, it may be that the family influence in this regard may stem largely from the model presented by the father. This is certainly a very tentative hypothesis, but one which seems worth investigating further.

When asked to associate to her boyfriend, she selects Design 7. The implication is that she may be transferring her focus of attention from her father to her boyfriend, possibly as representing a more satisfying relationship with a male figure.

Design 8 is indicated to be the one that the test subject associates with herself. This, too, suggests life dissatisfaction, as was hypothesized from her response to the least-liked design, and may therefore also be indicative of a poor self-concept. Study of the perceptual-motor performance in drawing this design, and consideration of her free-association to it, may help to support or clarify these interpretations.

Example Three: Adult Male, Married

Like Most?:   [IRT: 15"] Points to Design 3 and says, "I like the Christmas tree best."

Like Least?:   IRT: 58"] "It's almost a toss-up . . . I guess I would have to say . . . . I guess I would have to say the one with the picture and the crack in the wall" [a reference to associations made during the free-association phase]. Points to Design 4.

Mother?:   [IRT: 63"] "I guess the one with the eyes" [a reference to Design 8, but without pointing]. "My mother had almond-shaped eyes. They were . . . very large . . . very large.

Father?:   [IRT: 06"] Touches card bearing Design 3 and says, "The Christmas tree." Smiles.

Wife?:   [IRT: 46"] "You know what thought first struck my mind? Either this one," [points to Design 4], "or this one" [points to Design 5]. "But I didn't want to say it because this," [points to Design 4], "is the one I like the least . . . These two here" [points to Designs 4 and 5, respectively]. "These two seem to have more disorder than the others do, and I know she's not very organized. I'm sorry. I shouldn't have said that.

Self? : [IRT: 26"] "I don't know. I'd like to say . . . this one," [points to Design 3], "but . . . I guess this one" [points to Design 1].

Two general observations that immediately should stand out when considering the responses that have been made are (1) the relatively long delays between the presentation of most of the stimulus words and the associations that are made to them and (2) the relative wordiness of the test subject's verbalizations. This combination suggests the likelihood that the personality pattern of the individual is of the obsessive-compulsive type and that traits such as perfectionism and reflectiveness are characteristic of the individual.

Designating Design 3 as the one most liked suggests that ego-drive may be involved in the test subject's choice. Since the association is of Christmas, the indication is that his needs may tend to be child-like in nature. That his choice is prefaced by the words "I guess" implies a reluctance to assert himself unequivocally.

Internal conflict is indicated by the lengthy initial reaction time when asked to indicate his choice for the design which is least-liked. Equivocation and ambivalence are also revealed by words he uses such as *almost* and *toss-up*. Evidence that he possesses such traits is reflected once more in the words *I guess*, a term that he now uses repetitiously. Since the hesitance and disrupted fluency occur in connection with his association to Design 4, the hypothesis is that the trigger for what appear to be anxiety manifestations concerns the perceptions he has of his mother.

Support for the preceding hypothesis concerning the maternal connection is noted in his protracted initial reaction time when specifically asked to associate a design with *mother*. He again refers to a free-association, this time one he had made to Design 4 during the previous phase of the testing, which focuses on the image of his mother's eyes. This may be a projective indicator pointing to a memory of the mother figure as one whose watchfulness he was very aware of and to which he was very sensitive.

On the other hand, the directly elicited association to the stimulus word *father* indicates that the perception held of this significant other is far less anxiety-provoking than is true for the mother. This is inferred from the briefness of the initial reaction time, by the willingness to make physical contact with the stimulus card, and by the smile shown by the test subject when he responded. The link between the positive implications of the free-association to Design 3, "Christmas tree," and the selective-association to the stimulus word *father* seems to indicate that the perception of the father is a happy one.

When asked to identify a design with *wife*, internal conflict apparently is experienced once again, as suggested by the following observations: The initial reaction time increases, the test subject literally admits that he has conflicting thoughts, and he verbalizes awareness of the connection between what he previously associated with the least-liked design and the thought he has of his wife. His words, "struck me," when taken literally, imply the anticipation of hostile action or intent that may be directed against him, and hint at susceptibility to interpersonal anxiety. Since an initial hypothesis has suggested an obsessive-compulsive pattern in the test subject, the allusion to Design 4 and Design 5 as seeming to have "more disorder than the others do" and the reference to his wife as being "not very organized" may indicate awareness of a significant difference in the respective character styles of the respective spouses, a circumstance which may imply the existence of some marital dissatisfaction, if not difficulty. The tendency toward exaggerated superego development is theoretically consistent with the notion of the obsessive-compulsive personality pattern that is reflected in the guilt-laden self-reference, "I shouldn't have said that."

Attempting to associate one of the designs with himself appears to result in some confusion for the test subject. He first responds by saying, "I don't know," which not only may indicate uncertainty, but also may be an unconscious communication that repression is operating, the latter alternative suggesting that he is anxious about a view he holds of himself. He then indicates a wish to select Design 3 which he has previously identified as both the one most liked and the one that suggests *father* to him. That he rejects his apparent preference and designates Design 1 as the one to represent himself seems to indicate that, for some reason, he feels he should not make known the wish to identify with the father. This is possibly related to guilt about the respective differences he sees in the personalities of the two parents, a hypothesis that may be confirmed or refuted when a history is taken or when counseling is begun.

Example Four: Female Elementary School Child

Like Most? : "I like this one most." Picks up card bearing Design A and hands it to examiner. [Examiner accepts; then returns card to its place in the arrangement.]

Like Least? : Lowers head and, for first time during the administration, does not maintain eye contact with examiner. "I just don't like this one." Touches card bearing Design 5.

Mother? : Eye contact is resumed. "This one." Child picks up card bearing Design 4 and offers to examiner [Examiner accepts; then returns card to its place in the arrangement.]

Stepfather? : "This one." Points to Design 7 and says, "Because it's like the rocks" [a reference to the free-association previously elicited to Design 7.]

Teacher? : This one is my teacher one." Touches card bearing Design 1 and smiles.

Self? : "This one with the thing in the middle." Picks up card bearing Design 8 and offers to examiner.

By repeating the examiner's words as she responds to the first direction given her, this child is probably evidencing her desire to please authority figures. This also is suggested by her active motor-involvement in the task, that is, picking up the card and presenting it to the examiner. She has selected Design A as most liked, an indication that her relationship with the mother figure is probably a positive one.

Design 5 is identified as least-liked, suggesting that her experience in the home environment is perceived to be less than satisfactory. She does not parrot the examiners words this time, but makes the statement, "I just don't like this one." Using the word *just* in her verbalization, which on the surface would appear to be an unnecessary inclusion, may be a subtle communication that her feeling of not liking something is not a general attitude but one that is limited in its focus.

The test subject responds to the stimulus word *mother* by selecting Design A, again hinting at a strong connection with this parent. The resumption of eye-contact with the examiner suggests that her previous defensiveness has passed, a sign of good recoverability from intrapsychic stress.

When asked to associate to *stepfather*, she points to the card bearing Design 7, but avoids making physical contact with it. Given her tendency to pick up or make contact with each of the other cards, this avoidance seems significant and actually may represent a wish to avoid relating to her stepfather. Spontaneously commenting that she has selected this design because it was like the "rocks" perceived when reporting her free-association to Design 7 may indicate a perception of the stepfather as being difficult to relate to or as not being affectionate.

The test subject identifies Design 1 when asked which figure reminds her of her teacher. Her smile and the physical contact she makes with the stimulus card suggest that she has a satisfactory attitude toward this prominent person in her life. That this particular design is chosen may be an indication of the perception that a one-to-one relationship has been established between her and the teacher, or it may reflect the desire to establish such an individual relationship.

The selection of Design 8 as the one she associates with *self* suggests that the child is very aware of herself and her life space. Her calling attention to "the thing in the middle," a reference to the diamond within the hexagon, may be a projective communication that she sees herself as literally being in the "middle" of some life situation or set of circumstances. Given the preceding hypotheses, it seems reasonable to interpret this as the child calling attention to her perceived position in relationship to her mother on one side and her stepfather on the other, a matter that might profitably be explored in a parent interview.

ENDNOTES

1. The *Thematic Apperception Test* (Murray, 1943) is a projective technique which was originally designed to assist in the identification of *needs* (drive states) and *press* (environmental or external pressure). In the author's experience, it is particularly useful in obtaining information which may corroborate and amplify hypotheses that are developed through the use of the expanded approach to the Bender-Gestalt Test.

Chapter 7

PROJECTIVE ASSESSMENT
ILLUSTRATED

INTEGRATING THE PROJECTIVE DATA

As has been emphasized throughout this book, projective indicators of personality patterns and dynamics are to be found in abundance in the expanded approach to the Bender-Gestalt Test. Their occurrence, it has been shown, may take a variety of forms including visual, motoric, verbal, and nonverbal modes of expression, and it is in such separate categories that they have been presented and discussed. In actual clinical practice, however, the interpretive process is much more fluid and requires a deep appreciation of the unique ways in which response features occur in relation to one another. For example, when considering the drawing of Design 5, which is shown in Figure 44, the examiner must take into account a number of different observations in combination with each other in order to arrive at the most descriptive and applicable hypotheses about the test subject. The behavioral observations, of course, also must be considered in light of what is ascertained of the individual's life circumstances and history and, if known, the presenting problem on which a referral for psychological testing or counseling is based. It is the need for integration of the data from all available sources that is being accentuated here.

To illustrate how a basic hypothesis based on a projective sign may be broadened and enriched by integrating it with hypotheses derived from other projective signs, a discussion of the responses to one Bender-Gestalt design will be analyzed and interpreted. The information, observations, and hypotheses that follow are presented in the order in which they would be entertained and processed by the examiner who is conducting the projective assessment.

1. The test subject is a young adult male whose scholastic performance and athletic history throughout public school and private university have been consistently above-average. He presently holds the B.S. degree and operates a small, but successful retail business which he owns. His physical health is excellent and his medical history is benign. He is seeking counseling because he has noticed a gradual, but steady, decline in his motivation in general.

2. In the drawing of Design 5 (Figure 44), the gestalt is seen to be accurate, but the design slopes downward and circles are substituted for dots. Such perceptual-motor inaccuracies are not obvious in the other designs that he has drawn. The background of the individual suggests that cognitive development has been at least normal, and may be above-average, and there are no indications of physiological difficulties in the background information and history. He is certainly well above the age-expectancy for successful, i.e., accurate, reproduction of Design 5. The initial hypothesis, therefore, is that the perceptual-motor distortion can best be accounted for by personality factors, rather than organic or developmental ones.

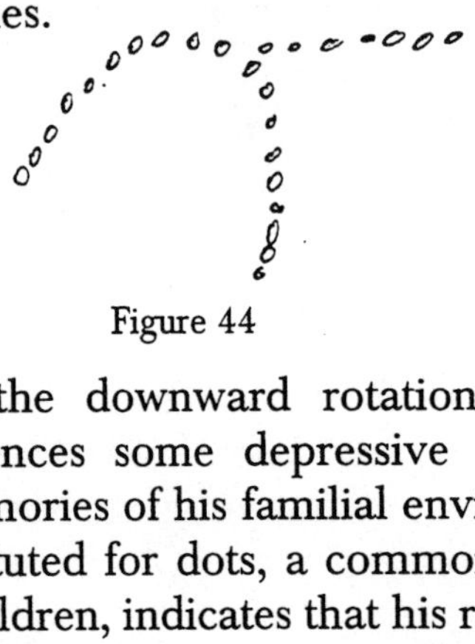

Figure 44

3. More specifically, the downward rotation suggests that the test subject experiences some depressive affect that is most likely related to memories of his familial environment.

4. Circles being substituted for dots, a common occurrence in the records of young children, indicates that his reactions to the family issues are likely to be immature in nature. It is reasonable to suspect that some fixation may have occurred in the personality's development.

5. It is also observed that the circles have been drawn with a light pencil pressure (the drawing is fainter than the others he has drawn). Since lightness of line is a feature occurring only in Design 5, the hypothesis is that although adequately secure in other areas of life, he tends to be timid when it comes to dealing with his family.

6. During the Free-Association Phase, the test subject responds as follows when presented with Design 5: "I don't know. It looks like a house, but it didn't turn out right. I don't know." Repeatedly saying, "I don't know," suggests that repression is operating in connection with thoughts or feelings about his experience of home, but also that whatever conflict does exist in this connection is strong enough to to be acknowledged, even if in an indirect fashion.

7. In the Selective-Association Phase, when asked which design is liked the least, he responds by touching the card bearing Design 5, saying, "I don't know why, but this one still isn't right." The selection of this design by the test subject reinforces the previously stated hypothesis about unresolved issues that pertain to his family, while his continued focus on the perception that the design "still isn't right" indicates that it is not only a past problem that is being communicated, but that the difficulties are affecting him even to this day.

8. Taken together, the projective interpretations indicate that the test subject is an individual who, consciously or unconsciously, harbors long-standing feelings and thoughts that may be pathogenic. From a mental health point of view, it seems both appropriate and clinically important to probe the matter with the individual, encourage him to deal with his issues in counseling, and to recognize that attempting to avoid them may result in future difficulties, for instance, in a family he someday may have of his own.

In this example, formulation of the initial hypothesis, i.e., that there is a psychological cause for the perceptual-motor irregularity, is only a beginning. It is amplified by considering many aspects of the test subject's response to this design, including the visual image he has drawn, the verbal associations elicited by the examiner, and the spontaneous verbalizations that were emitted as well. The available background information provides a tentative frame of reference from which to consider the potential significance of the observations made by the examiner during the test administration.

INTEGRATION: A CASE EXAMPLE

In discussing the integration of observational information and the hypotheses that may be generated from them, the focus of the preceding analysis was limited to the study of responses to a single design. Naturally, when working with the results of an administration in the clinical situation, *all* aspects of the test subject's response pattern will be considered. The examiner's interpretive approach, however, will be the same as modeled above, with emphasis being given to both the spontaneous and examiner-elicited verbal and nonverbal responses that occur before, during, and after the Traditional, Free-Association, and Selective-Association procedures have been administered. Again, the integration of the findings will be of paramount importance in the interpretive process. An example is given below.

Background

The test subject is an adolescent female who is in the tenth grade. She is reported by her guidance counselor to have scored in the superior range when administered a test of scholastic aptitude. Her schoolwork had been excellent through the sixth grade, but has been only marginally satisfactory beginning with her entrance into eighth grade. She has, at times, even received failing grades during some marking periods in high school despite her above-average performance on standardized achievement tests. She is described by her teachers as being quiet and usually uninvolved socially. Her parents have consistently refused to meet with school personnel to discuss their daughter, but they did agree to obtain psychological counseling for her after she was arrested for possession of a controlled substance and the recommendation for treatment was made by the court. There have been no medical difficulties in her history, and her physical development has been normative.

Rapport With The Examiner

The test subject's approach to the examiner was cooperative, subdued, with little spontaneity being shown. She spoke in a soft voice and usually did not make eye contact. Although she expressed indifference to the idea of counseling and a dislike for being tested, she agreed to participate in the administration of the Bender-Gestalt and did so compliantly.

The Traditional Procedure

The Bender-Gestalt designs drawn by the test subject are shown in Figure 45. They were completed in four minutes, twelve seconds.

The gestalts of the designs appear to be accurate and there are no errors of the type that are scoreable in most perceptual-motor diagnostic systems. Accuracy of perception may also be observed in the correct number of dots in Designs 1 and 3, columns and rows in Design 2, and curves in Design 6. Arrangement of the designs is orderly and suggests planning ability, but their concentration in the upper portion of the paper may reflect personality restriction and possibly the tendency to indulge in fantasy as a means of gratification or as a defense mechanism. The proximity of the drawings to each other may further reflect a tendency for the individual to be "closed," that is, unwilling to allow others to enter into her psychological space.

Design A

This drawing's most prominent features are the lightness of the lines and the workover of the entire square and the entire circle. Even the workover, however is done with very light pencil pressure so that all the lines appear to be faint. The lightness of line points to a hesitance of the test subject to express herself assertively to her mother, while the workover suggests that internal conflict and insecurity are strongly experienced in relation to her. The slightly open corner of the square at the point where it contacts the circle suggests the presence of immature dependency needs.

Design 1

In the case of this design, there is a noticeable increase in the boldness with which the drawing has been rendered, suggesting that she is likely to express herself more forcefully in an individual relationship. Given the insecurity hypothesized concerning the test subject's connection with her mother, it is tentatively hypothesized that she may have some other person or persons in her life to whom she can express herself and to whom she is likely to communicate with much less inhibition. Given the remarkable boldness with which the dots were executed, such expression may at times be in the form of ventilation. This hypothesis is also supported by the slight, but observable, upward slope in the line of dots, suggesting that in an individual interpersonal connection, she expresses herself outwardly rather than by turning inward or by acting shyly.

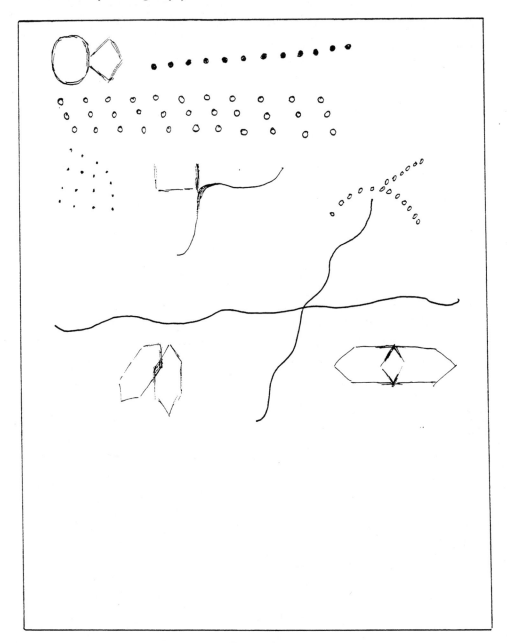

Figure 45

Design 2

Here, the design is drawn less boldly than was Design 1, but more so than was Design A. This suggests that adjustment in a group situation tends to be balanced and the behavior appropriate, as if the group norms provide a stabilizing influence for her. That she can function well, without either significant inhibition or excessive assertiveness, in a group setting is also indicated by the evenness and regularity of the rows and columns of circles, as well as by the absence of slope in this figure.

Design 3

Design 3 shows the correct number of dots and the correct number of angular elements. The last element is blunted, however, while the preceding elements show angles which decrease in sharpness as they are successively drawn from left to right. Projectively, this suggests that ego-drive has been progressively dampened or inhibited over time, and that while some goal-direction still is apparent in the test subject, its expression is not likely to be strongly apparent to others. It may also be observed that the length of the design (measured along its horizontal axis) is noticeably shorter than its length from from top to bottom with the result that the design appears to be compressed. This again suggests that ego-drive is being restrained and, in addition, that the personality undergoes some distortion as a consequence of that suppression, and the individual feels compelled to behave or present herself in ways other than she would prefer.

On the other hand, the entire design is sloped in an upward direction, a feature that is interpreted as suggestive of a tendency toward outward and impulsive self-expression. Although this would seem to contradict the previous notion of inhibition, the apparent difficulty can be reconciled by the hypothesis that the combination of signs pointing to inhibition on the one hand and acting-out on the other is indicative of a passive-aggressive solution to the problem posed by her need to express opposition to authority. This hypothesis would certainly be consistent with the reported pattern of academic underachievement shown by this intellectually-able adolescent.

Design 4

The manner in which Design 4 has been rendered is very similar to that of Design A. In both instances, the unusual features include lightness of line and workover, the latter being the result of retracing the movement of the pencil, but with little pencil pressure. Both of these designs, it will be remembered, share the hypothesis that the symbolic reference is likely to be that of the mother figure. Anxiety and insecurity are again strongly suggested. In addition, it is noted that the vertical dimensions of the open square are shorter than is depicted in the Bender-Gestalt stimulus figure, and there are gaps or breaks in the bottom line and at the corners of the square. The former feature is a projective indication that the test subject perceives the mother's capacity for nurturance to be limited; the latter feature suggests the experience of vulnerability in the relationship with the mother and an anticipated loss in the satisfaction of dependency needs.

Design 5

In the drawing of Design 5, circles are substituted for dots. The projective interpretation here is that the response to the familial environment is an immature one. The flattened appearance of the arc may indicate, as did the shortening of the sides of the square, that the family is perceived as limited as a resource for the satisfaction of emotional needs. This flattening may also be a reflection of the pressure she feels to inhibit self-expression, and may constitute support for the similar hypothesis formulated when the flattening or compression effect observed in Design 3 was considered.

Design 6

This design reproduction is of special interest because it is larger than the others and it stands alone on the horizontal plane on which it was drawn. It is also placed at the center between the paper's right and left margins. These combined indicators appear to signal the test subject's personal identification with this particular design, which in turn suggests that something of central importance to her is being projectively expressed. Since the sinusoidal curves are clearly flattened, it may be that this is a communication about the depressed state that she is experiencing, and that she is very preoccupied with the dysphoric affect. It may also be observed that the upper extension of the vertical wavy line enters into the concave area of the arc of Design 5. The hypothesis suggested by this combination of features is that the test subject associates the depression or sadness she feels with the circumstances of her family situation.

Design 7

The drawing of Design 7 shows very good integration of the two hexagons, again testifying to the test subject's perceptual-motor competence. The lines, however, are faintly drawn and there is workover at the point where the hexagons overlap. These signs lead to the hypothesis that, as in the relationship with the mother, considerable anxiety and conflict are experienced in connection with the father figure. Similarly, the small gaps which may be noted in the lines and at the junctures of the angles of the hexagons suggest some feelings of vulnerability in the relationship and a fear of loss of impulse control.

Design 8

In the last design reproduction, the lines of the hexagon are very lightly drawn. There is also workover present immediately above and below the inner diamond. These features suggest that considerable anxiety is felt by the test subject in connection with the way she sees herself in her life space, and particularly in connection with how she experiences the restraints that are imposed on her by the world. The upper and lower points of the central diamond are drawn more boldly and actually penetrate the hexagon where contact is made with it. Projectively, this is seen as a representation of the test subject's effort to penetrate or break through the limits that she feels are imposed on her from without. That it is only the points, and not the entire diamond, that have been drawn with heavy pencil pressure is an indication that there is some reluctance felt concerning the ego-drive she is attempting to express.

Tentative Conclusions: Traditional Procedure

The test subject appears to be an insecure and anxiety-prone individual with unresolved dependency needs. She is probably unhappy about her life circumstances and fails to find emotional support in the relationship she has with her parents. She would like to assert her individuality, but is hesitant to do so directly and probably resorts to passive-aggressive means to express her frustration and any hostility she experiences. She probably can find support in a one-to-one social relationship where she may feel comparatively safe to act-out her impulses. When in a group situation, she is likely to be influenced by its standards, and probably will behave in a more conforming manner.

The Free-Association Procedure

Design A   IRT: 19"

Association: I saw it as two people. I can't explain it. I wish I could.

Interpretation: Conflict and uncertainty are suggested by the prolonged initial reaction time, while confusion is indicated by the statement, "I can't explain it." The desire to understand is implied by her final utterance, "I wish I could."

Design 1   IRT: 07"

Association: "This is a very enlarged line of dots that you can put your signature on."

Interpretation: Here, the shorter initial reaction time suggests that the test subject is demonstrating more self-confidence. The idea of a signature suggests that she is identifying herself, possibly because she experiences greater safety when thinking of herself in an individual relationship.

Design 2   IRT: 05"

Association: "People marching . . . in a parade . . . but they need to line up a little bit better."

Interpretation: This appears to be an expression of conformity and the pressure to follow the group. In the same vein, "marching" implies that orders are being followed, but the possibility of some passive-aggressive resistance is also hinted at by the comment that". . . they need to line up a little bit better."

Design 3   IRT: 12"

Association: "Sound waves." (Q) "Like they're bouncing off something."

Interpretation: Projectively, this suggests a need to communicate or, perhaps, to be heard. Her words, "bouncing off something," may indicate that the test subject feels that she is not being heard by others.

Design 4   IRT: 21"

Association: "They don't match very well." (Q) "I don't know what they are . . . They just don't seem to match."

Interpretation: Conflict and inability to relate to the mother are suggested by the failure to produce a specific association and by the insistence that the two design elements are not a match. The relatively extended initial reaction time also is suggestive of intrapsychic conflict that involves maternal issues.

Design 5   IRT: 07"

Association: "An igloo that's being squashed, with something trying to get out."

Interpretation: Use of *igloo* is an indication that the home environment is perceived as emotionally cold. The experience of external pressure is connoted by the action, "being squashed." Since the test subject uses the present tense in her verbal description, the implication is that a current condition is being described. "Trying to get out" is interpreted projectively as an expression of the desire to escape from the restrictiveness she perceives in connection with her family

Design 6   IRT: 15"

Association: "Nothing." (Q) "Nothing. No . . . Nothing."

Interpretation: This is a rejection and implies an inability or an unwillingness to deal with the symbolism of the design and the associations that consciously or unconsciously are being evoked. Projectively, it may be an indication of the test subject's need to deny how unhappy or depressed she is.

Design 7   IRT: 11"

Association: "Two people who are separate . . . but could be together."

Interpretation: The test subject is probably expressing her awareness that the relationship with her father is not close. She also seems to imply that she perceives the possibility of some improvement.

Design 8   IRT: 09"

Association: "Eye." (Q) "Just an eye. It also could be like a traffic sign." (Q) "A stop sign . . . but sort of squashed."

Interpretation: The initial association is "Eye."   This actually is a homonym since it may refer either to the visual organ or the pronoun *I*. The punning aspect is made more emphatic because the test subject does not preface the word with the indefinite article, *an,* the use of which would have made her intention more clear. When the examiner inquires, however, she responds by using the article, ostensibly indicating that she means *eye*. Nevertheless, the clinical implication is that she may be projectively indicating that this Bender-Gestalt design, and her verbal association to it, are references to herself. That the self-identification she appears to be acknowledging in the free-association also applies to the non-verbal projections that have been noted in her drawing of the design is supported by the consistency of the themes in each instance: They relate to the experience of external or environmental pressure to restrain self-expression. The present verbal associations include a "stop sign" which symbolizes external control or the need for restraint. The traffic sign being seen as "squashed" is a further indication of the extent of the pressure to conform to external rules and the expectations of others.

Tentative Conclusions: Free-Association Procedure

The projective evidence indicates that the test subject is reacting to perceived pressure to conform to the values and expectations of others, particularly her parents. This pressure is perceived by her as excessive. She is frustrated and unhappy, and feels affectionally deprived in her family situation. She is also confused about her relations with her parents, particularly the mother, and has unsatisfied dependency needs. When in a group situation, she probably will inhibit self-expression unless such expression is consistent with the standards she believes would be acceptable to the other members.

The Selective-Association Procedure

Like Most?:   Points to Design 1 with index finger. "It's simple." (Q) "Not complicated." (Q) "The design."

Like Least?:   "This one." Taps Design 5 with index finger.

Mother?:   "Mother? That's hard . . . Maybe this one." Points to Design 4 with index finger.

Father?:   "This one." Points to Design 8 with index finger.

Self?:   Touches Design 3 with index finger.

School?:   "This one." Touches Design 2 with index finger.

In selecting the design liked the most, the test subject makes the comment, "It's simple." Because it is not clear whether she is referring to the task, the design, or both, an inquiry becomes necessary. Her response, "Not complicated," fails to clarify the matter, so she is questioned again, and this time she indicates that it is the design to which she refers. The interpretation of her choice of the words "simple" and "uncomplicated" is that she is expressing a wish for her life to be easier, implying that it is not already perceived to be that way. Since the most-liked design is hypothesized to reflect one's attitude toward individual relationships, it may be that it is in the one-to-one connection that she believes relief from turmoil is to be found.

Design 5 is chosen as the least-liked of the series. This is suggestive of dissatisfaction with her familial connection, a hypothesis which supports the interpretations of emotional coldness and parental pressure which were posited earlier.

When asked to identify a design with her mother, the test subject repeats the stimulus word and says, "That's hard." This suggests that conflict is experienced in connection with that parent who may be seen as rigid or unfeeling. Her free-association to this figure, it may be recalled, was blocked and all she was did was to acknowledge a sense that the two design elements failed to match one another.

The test subject's next selective-association is direct and not elaborated. She identifies Design 8 with her father. This suggests that she may perceive her father as the main source of the pressure she experiences to conform or to meet parental standards and it may be primarily the father with whom she feels herself to be in a power struggle.

Responding only nonverbally, the test subject indicates that Design 3 is the one she associates with herself. The absence of verbalization may reflect defensiveness and an intent to avoid revealing herself. It also may be a hint that she is depressed about what this design consciously or unconsciously symbolizes for her, namely the thwarting of the expression of her individuality.

The last selective-association elicited is to the stimulus word *school.* Here she selects Design 2. This may be interpreted as an expression of the test subject's view of school as as a place of conformity. The absence of spontaneous remarks, combined with the observations that this design was less boldly drawn than was Design 1, and that the reproduction did not reveal any projective indicator of acting-out, suggests that it is unlikely that she will be a behavior problem in the school setting.

Tentative Conclusions: Selective-Association Procedure

The projective hypotheses that result from an analysis of the test-subject's responses to this phase of the testing again point to dependence-independence issues, the experience of pressure to conform or to live up to external standards, and the deprivation of affectional needs. She appears to experience her mother as emotionally inaccessible and her father as the power against whom she may have to assert herself. She probably will appear to be conforming and nontroublesome in formal group situations such as school.

The projective hypotheses that have been developed in connection with this portion of the multiphase Bender-Gestalt administration are supportive of, and consistent with, those previously derived from the analysis of the designs which were drawn by the test subject and the associations that were elicited in connection with them.

Additional Interpretive Hypotheses

Understanding of this adolescent may be increased through the generation of propositional psychological interpretations (Murstein,

1965) which may be applicable. For instance, since the hypotheses already generated suggest that the test subject longs to express her individuality, but that she is largely unable to do so directly or assertively, it is reasonable to anticipate that if she does express opposition to the restrictiveness she believes is imposed on her, she would be likely to do so in an indirect manner, for example, through passive-aggressive behavior, a conclusion that is consistent with specific projective interpretations made earlier. The adoption of such a response pattern, of course, would be quite consistent with the school's perception of her as a bright underachiever.

Another propositional interpretation may be considered. This would be in response to the hypothesized meaning that a one-to-one relationship signifies for this test subject. In the drawing of Figure 1, it was observed that there is an upward slope to the boldly drawn line of dots, this combination of features suggesting an inclination to express her impulses outwardly when in an individual relationship. In the Free-Association Procedure, it seems as if she is unconsciously acknowledging her personal identification with the importance that the symbolism of Design 1 holds for her, e.g., ". . . a line of dots that you can put your signature on." Similarly, during the Selective-Association Procedure, she identifies Design 1 as the design that is most liked, and justifies her choice by alluding to it as "uncomplicated."

Taken together these observations suggest the *possibility* that this girl may already have established an important personal relationship with a particular person whose existence has not yet been disclosed to parents or counselor, but with whom she is able to express herself more assertively. One might even wonder if it is in this connection that she has become involved with marijuana use. While the very speculative nature of these possibilities makes it inappropriate to include them in a psychological report, they would nevertheless be of potentially great relevance and therefore would be very important to explore in the confidentiality of a counseling relationship.

Chapter 8

APPLICATIONS IN COUNSELING AND PSYCHOTHERAPY

INTRODUCTION

During the years since the Bender-Gestalt Test first appeared on the diagnostic scene, its primary use has been as an instrument for the evaluation of perceptual-motor functioning. As such, it has helped the clinician in the identification of some types of neurological impairment and it has been shown to be an effective means of assessing children's developmental maturity and readiness for school learning. It also has been thought of, and utilized as, a projective method for the purpose of revealing the more subjective and unconscious aspects of personality functioning and dynamics.

In the current book, a method has been offered that broadens the scope of the projective application of the Bender-Gestalt by requiring the test subject to respond verbally, as well as nonverbally, to the stimulus designs. By expanding the screen on which the subject can project the marks of his or her individuality for consideration and interpretation by the examiner, the clinical information that may be gleaned about the individual is greatly increased.

In addition to its demonstrated diagnostic utility, however, the Bender-Gestalt Test, especially when used in conjunction with the multiphase method of administration, will be found to serve other clinical purposes as well. It may also be used, for instance, as a practical device that can facilitate both the clinician's and the client's work in counseling and psychotherapy.

As stated earlier, the effectiveness of the Bender-Gestalt Test in evaluating the presence of perceptual-motor anomalies, and their implications for organicity, has been well-established both in research and in clinical practice. In this chapter, however, the author's aim is to discuss the versatility of the Bender-Gestalt Test as a psychological tool of *wider* relevance by describing some of its less traditional applications, particularly in the areas of counseling and psychotherapy. Such a presentation is felt to be justified for at least two reasons:

1. The administration of the expanded technique is simple and often can be accomplished in as little as ten minutes time. Given the extensive caseloads carried by most psychotherapists and counselors, simplicity and brevity make it less stressful an experience for test subject and examiner alike.

2. The Bender-Gestalt Test is already widely-used in many professional contexts. Many psychologists who work in schools and learning centers, for instance, will routinely use the Bender-Gestalt, or a similar measure, as part of the diagnostic battery needed to conduct psychoeducational assessments. The ability to use the *same* test to obtain *more diverse* information about the test subject is obviously both economically and procedurally advantageous.

CLINICAL DIAGNOSIS

While the formulation of a clinical diagnosis, e.g., determining a DSM-IV Axis I or Axis II classification (American Psychiatric Association, 1994) for a given client, is an important part of the helping process, it is in itself not a sufficient basis for choosing the specific type of treatment or remediation that should be employed. Nor does a clinical diagnosis necessarily indicate the particular life issues actually being faced by the individual or the manner he or she is likely to adopt in responding to those issues (Weiner, 1975). Nevertheless, information concerning such variables must be garnered and understood in order to establish an appropriate treatment focus and to develop a balanced and comprehensive treatment plan. In counseling and psychotherapy, for example, there are many understandings that are necessary for guiding therapeutic interaction and suggesting the relevant aspects of personality that would be most advantageous to explore. Such understandings relate to client characteristics or circumstances such as the following:

1. *Direction and strength of drives.* These include motivations such as sexual, aggressive, affiliative, competitive, etc., and their respective strengths.

2. *Preoccupations.* This refers to what the immediate and long-term focus of attention might be, i.e., what the individual has on his or her mind.

3. *Moods and emotions that are being experienced.* Included here are feelings and moods being experienced by the individual, as well as the degree to which they are under intellectual control.

4. *Comfort in social situations in general.* This refers to the tendency to move into or away from participation with individuals, groups, or both, and may reflect attitudes toward gender, age, authority, and similar identifiers of others.

5. *Attitudes toward significant others in particular.* This includes perceptions of specific persons to whom the individual desires, or is required, to relate such as parents, spouse, boss, teacher, etc.

It is its wonderful suitability as a device for eliciting cues that may be used to generate hypotheses concerning these variables that makes the multiphase approach to the Bender-Gestalt Test so helpful clinically. It has been explained that in attempting to reproduce the stimulus designs, the test subject will communicate nonverbally his or her conscious and unconscious inclinations and personal meanings through the introduction of specific features or deviations in the drawings. How the separate elements of a design are drawn in relation to one another, for instance, is projectively suggestive of the attitudes, feelings, and behaviors whose presence can be anticipated in the test subject's actual interpersonal relations. In the same way, verbal communications, both spontaneous and examiner-elicited, provide the opportunity for the examiner to "hear" parallel communications whose symbolic expression allows them to bypass the test subject's ego-censorship. Equipped with such insights early in the helping process allows the counselor or therapist to evaluate the extent to which issues are being faced or avoided by a client, and to observe the types of defenses and coping skills that are characteristically used to deal with them.

Beside arriving at the initial diagnostic formulation, the psychological examiner will often find it useful to conduct a personality assessment well after the commencement of treatment. This may be for the purpose of developing understanding of the client's current dynamics and especially his or her unconscious preoccupations at this later time during the treatment process. Retesting can also shed light on the extent to which growth, as reflected in affective and cognitive changes suggested by present test performance, may have taken place. As has already been stated, one of the advantages of using the Bender-Gestalt, in this case for reevaluation, is that it can be done so quickly and conveniently during the treatment session, i.e., without using all or most of the clinical hour for that purpose.

THE BENDER-GESTALT AS A TEACHING DEVICE

One of the applications of the expanded approach to the Bender-Gestalt Test that the author has found to be particularly useful and gratifying involves guiding the counseling or psychotherapy client to learn what the test may reveal about personality. The purposes here are several:

First, in developing a treatment plan, more than the presenting problem will need to be considered. For example, while the client may be seeking a specific outcome as a result of treatment, there may be additional, and often more important, therapeutic goals that should be considered by him or her, but which have not been articulated or even recognized as relevant. A person who comes to a counselor because of a wish to overcome a specific phobia, for instance, may not have insight into the significant internal or external variables that play a part in the development of that symptom. Helping the individual to identify the actual circumstances which may be etiologically significant is often facilitated by bringing them into focus through a discussion of what the Bender-Gestalt Test responses seem to indicate. This is particularly likely to be so when the free-associations and the selective-associations are read back to the client and discussed one after another. Frequently, the internal consistency that will be found in the hypotheses generated from those associations, plus exploration of the *new* associations that will inevitably be made by the client when discussing his or her original associations, will serve to jell in the mind of the client the issues that will be appropriate to deal with if the therapeutic goals are to be reached.

Second, the discussion of the client's responses to the test, when sequentially reviewed, provide needed opportunity to support, confirm, and extend projective interpretations of the type that have been modeled in this book. This is almost always beneficial, not only to the client, but to the counselor (who presumably also has been the psychological examiner) as well. In the case of the client, he or she begins to go through a process of desensitization as the relevant life issues are repeatedly brought into focus by the skillful presentations of the counselor. In addition, the author has found that the client invariably develops a higher degree of appreciation for the knowledge and skill that the counselor is perceived as possessing, the result usually being a heightened sense of optimism about being guided through the treatment process. In the case of the examiner, especially one who is just beginning to employ the projective approach to diagnosis and treatment, there will be opportunity for abundant reinforcement of the accuracy and utility of the projective hypotheses that have been generated. Even for experienced projectively-oriented examiners and counselors, the appreciation for the ubiquitousness of projective communication and its value as a means of understanding self and others can continue to expand.

Third, by guiding the client in the interpretation of his or her own responses, skills and attitudes are being developed that will be of help not only in the treatment context, but in life in general. The client is helped to learn that by paying attention to what is being communicated through the projective process, one is able to discern the needs that are present, but that previously may not have been attended to or perhaps even recognized. With such recognition, the range of choices available to the individual may be broadened and the assuming of responsibility for making the most appropriate ones may be enhanced.

REFERENCES

Abt, E. L., & Bellak, L. (Eds.). (1950). *Projective psychology*. New York: Alfred A. Knopf.

American Psychiatric Association. (1994). *Diagnostic and statistical manual of mental disorders* (4th ed.). Washington, D.C. Author.

Bender, L. (1938). *A visual motor gestalt test and its clinical use*. New York: American Orthopsychiatric Association.

Clawson, A. (1962). *The Bender Visual-motor Gestalt Test for children: A manual*. Los Angeles: Western Psychological Services.

Combs, A. W., & Snygg, D. (1959). *Individual behavior: A perceptual approach to behavior*. New York: Harper & Brothers.

Frank, L. K. (1948). *Projective methods*. Springfield, IL: Charles C Thomas.

Gilbert, J. (1978) *Interpreting psychological test data*. New York: Van Nostrand Reinhold.

Hammer, E. (1981). *The clinical application of projective drawings.* Springfield, IL: Charles C Thomas.

Jung, C. G. (1954). *The development of personality.* Princeton, NJ: Princeton University Press.

Jung, C. G. (1966). *The practice of psychotherapy* (2nd ed.). Princeton, NJ: Princeton University Press.

Jung, C. G. (1971). *Psychological types.* Princeton, NJ: Princeton University Press.

Klatskin, E. H., McNamara, N. E., Shaffer, D., & Pincus, J. (1972). Minimal organicity in children of normal intelligence: Correspondence between psychological test results and neurological findings. *Journal of Learning Disabilities, 5,* 213-218.

Koppitz, E. M. (1962), Diagnosing brain damage in young children with the Bender Gestalt Test. (1962). *Journal of Consulting Psychology, 26,* 541-546.

Koppitz, E. M. (1964). *The Bender-Gestalt Test for young children.* New York: Grune & Stratton.

Koppitz, E. M. (1975). *The Bender Gestalt Test for young children. Volume II. Research and applications. 1963-1973.* Needham Heights, MA: Allyn and Bacon.

Kramer, E., & Fenwick, J. (1966). Differential diagnosis with the Bender Gestalt Test. *Journal of Projective Techniques and Personality Assessment, 30,* 59-61.

Lacks, P. (1984). *Bender Gestalt screening for brain dysfunction.* New York: Wiley.

Lacks, P., & Newport, K. (1980). A comparison of scoring systems and level of scorer experience on the Bender Gestalt Test. *Journal of Personality Assessment, 44,* 351-357.

Lerner, E. A. (1972). *The projective use of the Bender Gestalt.* Springfield, IL: Charles C Thomas.

Murray, H. A. (1943) *Thematic Apperception Test.* Cambridge, MA: Harvard University Press.

Murstein, B. I. (Ed.). (1965). *Theory and research in projective techniques (Emphasizing the TAT).* New York: Basic Books.

Ogdon, D. P. (1975). *Psychodiagnostics and personality assessment: A handbook* (2nd ed.). Los Angeles, CA: Western Psychological Services.

Pascal, G. R., & Suttell, B. J. (1951). *The Bender-Gestalt Test.* New York: Grune & Stratton.

Perticone, E. X., & Tembeckjian, R. M. (1987). *The mosaic technique in personality assessment: A practical guide.* Rosemont, NJ: Programs for Education.

Phillips, L., & Smith, J. G. (1953). *Rorschach interpretation: Advanced technique.* New York: Grune & Stratton.

Reik, T. (1956). *Listening with the third ear: The inner experience of a psychoanalyst.* New York: Grove Press.

Sarason, S. B., Davidson, K. S., Lighthall, F. F., Waite, R. R., & Ruebush, B. K. (1960). *Anxiety in elementary school children.* New York: Wiley.

Tolor, A., & Brannigan, G. G. (1980). *Research and clinical applications of the Bender-Gestalt test.* Springfield, IL: Charles C Thomas.

Tolor, A., & Schulberg, H. (1963). *An evaluation of the Bender-Gestalt Test.* Springfield, IL: Charles C Thomas.

Weiner, I. B. (1975). *Principles of psychotherapy.* New York: Wiley.

Yonda, A. J. (1984). *Popular verbal associations to the Bender Visual-Motor Gestalt Test.* Unpublished master's thesis, State University of New York at Oswego, Oswego, NY.

INDEX